DISCARD

THE SURGERY-FREE
MAKEOVER

THE SURGERY-FREE MAKEOVER

*All You Need to Know for Great Skin
and a Younger Face*

BRANDITH IRWIN, M.D.

Da Capo

LIFE
LONG

A MEMBER OF THE PERSEUS BOOKS GROUP

Designed by Lesley Rock for SquareOne Publishing Partners
Set in 12.5 point Arno Pro Display by Lesley Rock for SquareOne Publishing Partners
Illustrations by Neal Rohrer

Library of Congress Cataloging-in-Publication Data
Irwin, Brandith, 1952–
    The surgery-free makeover : all you need to know for great skin and a younger face / Brandith Irwin. — 1st Da Capo Press ed.
        p.   cm.
    Includes bibliographical references and index.
    ISBN 978-0-7382-1118-3 (alk. paper)
    1. Skin—Care and hygiene. 2. Beauty, Personal. 3. Women—Health and hygiene. I. Title.
RL87.I793 2008
646.7'2—dc22

                                                                                    2008014602

First Da Capo Press edition 2008

Published by Da Capo Press
A Member of the Perseus Books Group
www.dacapopress.com

Note: The information in this book is true and complete to the best of our knowledge. This book is intended only as an informative guide for those wishing to know more about health issues. In no way is this book intended to replace, countermand, or conflict with the advice given to you by your own physician. The ultimate decision concerning care should be made between you and your doctor. We strongly recommend you follow his or her advice. Information in this book is general and is offered with no guarantees on the part of the authors or Da Capo Press. The authors and publisher disclaim all liability in connection with the use of this book. The names and identifying details of people associated with events described in this book have been changed. Any similarity to actual persons is coincidental.

Da Capo Press books are available at special discounts for bulk purchases in the U.S. by corporations, institutions, and other organizations. For more information, please contact the Special Markets Department at the Perseus Books Group, 2300 Chestnut Street, Suite 200, Philadelphia, PA, 19103, or call (800) 810-4145, extension 5000, or e-mail special.markets@perseusbooks.com.

10 9 8 7 6 5 4 3 2 1

CONTENTS

INTRODUCTION

The calendar and the mirror may say forty or fifty, but the spirit inside you says thirty, maybe thirty-five. Should you accept the changes in your face and accept that one day you'll look like your mother? Not the women I know. How about plastic surgery? Too risky, too expensive, and you're too young anyway. Maybe when you're sixty.

I'm convinced that almost every woman on the other side of forty has three or four things she'd like to change about her face. But how can you do it safely, effectively, and economically? What if you have a class reunion coming up? A wedding? An important work event? What if you're on a budget? How can you make the best decisions for your skin, your face, your time, and your budget?

Women in their forties, fifties, and sixties know we can't get away with doing nothing anymore. And we also know that the creams that promise so much aren't really going to repair the problems we see. Perhaps you're bothered by frown lines, upper-lip lines, crow's feet, lines around the mouth, baggy eyelid skin, loose skin around the jawline, or sun damage on your chest. If you need a plan to get your youngest face, read on. This book will give you the tools to look your vibrant best.

In my practice, nearly every woman (or man) I talk to about her (or his) skin is overwhelmed by the number of products and the wealth of information available. Today thousands of skin-care products and dozens of lasers, peels, and injectables are easily at hand, while cosmetic companies, laser, and injectable manufacturers spend millions of dollars to promote the latest new cream or technology. It's no wonder today's woman has trouble figuring out what works.

In this book, I'll give you the key information you'll need to "fix your face." We'll take a tour of your face, and I'll show you along the way what

1

you can fix and how. I'll give you timelines for events and different skin plans for different budgets. Most important, I'll help you set up a realistic plan.

If you're anything like the patients I've treated over the past fifteen years, you expect treatments to be a good value for your money, whether that's three hundred dollars or ten thousand dollars. You also expect your treatments to be safe and hope they'll require minimum time out of your busy schedule. Moreover, you want products that'll work *for you.* The average woman has dozens of products cluttering her bathroom drawers. Just think of how many expensive products you've purchased in the past five years that promised to work miracles but didn't? How many have given you allergic or irritant reactions? Let's be honest: it's an awful lot of time and trouble to return those ineffective products for a refund.

After reading this book, you should feel as though you've had a personal skin consultation that helps you to focus on the areas of your face that you'd most like to improve. You should also feel better armed to discuss with your own doctor, nurse, or aesthetician the treatments or products that will help you. Finding the right doctor, and having a good relationship with him or her, can make all the difference in developing your own skin plan for the future.

GETTING STARTED—YOUR SKIN PLAN

When my patients come in for a consultation, they generally want to leave with a *plan* for their makeover. Usually they know exactly what's bothering them, whether it's frown lines, crow's feet, lines around the mouth, or some sagging at the jawline. But often they don't know how to get from where they are to *where they want to be.* That's where cosmetic dermatologists like myself come in.

My goal is to help you figure out how to get from A to B with a plan that covers the areas you want to fix within your budget and your time frame. From products that help prevent problems in the first place, to

Botox and fillers, to lasers and radiofrequency, to maintaining your skin, you can create your own skin makeover.

Our skin is a part of us. That may sound obvious, but if we're not healthy and vibrant, our skin won't be. I don't believe in aging gracefully—I believe in aging vigorously—in other words—with intention, vitality, and vigor. Much of aging is just disuse and misuse, whether it's sun-damaged skin, an alcohol-damaged liver, or deteriorating joints from too much or too little exercise.

In four simple steps, you can use the chapters in this book to help you. First, as with most of my patients, I'd encourage you to think about the three things that you'd most like to change about your face. They might be frown lines, lines on your upper lip, brown spots or age spots, lines from the nose to mouth, or sagging at the jawline.

Second, as you read through, keep a working list of what can be done about each individual problem as you come across it. For instance, you might be worrying about wrinkles around the eyes. We'll discuss the various products and procedures, from eye creams to Botox to CosmoDerm, as potential solutions.

If you're worried that you don't have deep pockets for expensive procedures, know that many of the plans and procedures suggested in this book are affordable, even on a strict budget. Sometimes it's simply a matter of rechanneling money you might otherwise spend on worthless products or unhelpful procedures onto procedures appropriate for your skin. When possible, I've outlined a range of prices for various cosmetic services. Please bear in mind, though, that costs vary from place to place. You'll likely pay more in New York or Los Angeles, for instance, for the same procedure in Omaha or Portland.

Third, keep track of what it will cost you to correct each problem with its accompanying solution: for instance, you might note that you want to fix your crow's feet. With a better moisturizer, you'll pay around sixty dollars; if you go for Botox, your out-of-pocket expense will more likely be around four hundred dollars. What's more feasible for your budget?

Fourth and finally, by the time you finish the book, you should have a sense of the timeline for addressing each of your problem areas. Is it a matter of a one-time visit to a cosmetic dermatologist or multiple visits stretched out over a few months or a year? What does your schedule allow? Are you looking for more of a quick fix? These are all questions to keep in mind as you formulate your skin plan going forward.

Toward the book's end, I offer plenty of advice on how to find a good cosmetic dermatologist and laser center in your area and guide you on the kinds of questions to ask to ensure you're signing up with a safe and reliable doctor. Once you've formulated your skin plan for your trouble areas, you'll need a maintenance plan—a plan to keep your youngest face looking its best. After all, you don't spend time and energy to remodel a house only to let it fall into disrepair!

But before you begin, take the Quiz for Your Skin below.

See how healthy or sun damaged your skin is now. Taking the quiz will help you answer the question, How is my skin doing?

1. Is your skin color:
   A. Even and one color throughout.
   B. A few brown or red spots here and there.
   C. Lots of brown or red blotches.
   D. I feel like my face looks like a pizza on a good day.
2. Any sagging?
   A. I'm under thirty.
   B. Very little and when I pinch my skin, it bounces back quickly.
   C. I have some sagging around the jaw line and my upper neck.
   D. I definitely have jowls, and my neck is a problem.
3. Any wrinkles?
   A. None at rest or smiling.
   B. Only when I smile.
   C. I can see wrinkles around my eyes and around my mouth even when I'm not smiling.
   D. I have wrinkles all over.

4. I feel like I look

    A.   Rested and healthy.

    B.   Good, but like I've had a little too much sun.

    C.   I definitely have some problem areas.

    D.   Tired and older than most of my friends.

Give yourself 0 for every A answer, 1 for every B answer, 2 for every C, and 3 for every D.

If you scored **zero to 2,** that's fabulous. You can focus mainly on prevention and maintenance.

If you scored **3 to 6,** that's also very good. You probably need just a little bit of repair and then to focus on a good maintenance regimen. You could also focus on a particular area, like your crow's feet area or your lips.

If you scored **7 to 12,** you will definitely want to consider some repair work to fix the damage that's already been done and then go on to a more effective maintenance regimen.

Remember, it's never too late to take care of your skin, even if you're sixty or sixty-five years old with significant sun damage. Most of what we think of as normal aging in skin is really *not* normal aging. It's too much sun, unhealthy lifestyles, and environmental damage. But we now have

- excellent products,
- gentle lasers to correct brown spots and red blotchiness,
- new skin-tightening lasers to reduce sagging skin, and
- injections to relax or fill out wrinkles.

With this book to help you, you can do a lot without plastic surgery to return your face to its wrinkle-free and glowing birthright!

PART ONE
AN OVERVIEW
Products, Procedures, and More

1

WONDERFULLY SCENTED, EVER-TEMPTING PRODUCTS

Give a woman a fish and you feed her for a day; but teach a woman to fish and you feed her for a lifetime.
—*Anonymous*

I know you want me to just cut through all the confusion and tell you what products to use to get the face you want. That would help you for a few weeks or months, until the seasons change, until you go on vacation to a different climate, or until your hormones trigger a change in your skin's oil production. But it won't help you over the long term because you and the products keep changing. I would rather teach you how to *think* about products, so you won't waste any more time and money on them unnecessarily.

But first. There are good reasons we women like products! If we understand what we want from products, we'll have a better chance of buying the right ones for the right reasons. Here are some of those reasons:

- Products are a small slice of daily self-care that doesn't take a lot of time from our busy schedules. Taking five to ten minutes morning and night to care for our skin represents a little time for ourselves.
- They are sensual—the packaging is beautiful, and they smell and feel good.

- They're affordable luxuries—like caramel lattes. We may not be able to afford that five-hundred-dollar handbag, but that forty-dollar moisturizer could be a treat.
- They can make our skin look better—let's not overlook the obvious!
- They're part of the communal language of women—like sports for some men. We understand and talk about these things with each other.
- They can represent hope—we know in our hearts that the implied promise of looking better and maybe younger might not happen—but we can always hope.

But many women today are in the throes of what I like to call product insanity. When you multiply the number of products available (approximately forty thousand) by the number of places to buy those different products (department stores, Internet, etc.), there are approximately 320,000 choices to make about what to buy and where to buy it. Who can possibly track this amount of information accurately?

And then there are all the different product categories, such as cleansers, toners, sunscreens, moisturizers, repair creams, eye creams, lightening creams, acne creams, oil control products, and more.

In this chapter, I recommend those tried and true products that have some solid science and a track record behind them. I and many of my patients have used many of these for years. But I can't personally try every product out there, and I know there are good ones that I've missed. So, if you have some great ones that are working for you, stick with them!

WHICH PRODUCTS DO YOU *REALLY* NEED?

When you're reading about cleansers, moisturizers, and toners, keep in mind that each of us has an individual skin type. You may have to try several different products before you find one that you really like and that agrees with your skin. We all have different reactions to fragrances, the feel of a cream, or even the color of it.

Still, that said, there are some good general rules about ingredients to keep in mind when considering beauty products:

- Avoid products that list any kind of alcohol in the first five ingredients.
- Avoid products with long lists of ingredients—the fewer ingredients, the better.
- If you are "sensitive," avoid products with plant extracts and fragrance. Try the Free & Clear line.
- The term *noncomedogenic* ("doesn't cause acne") may be helpful, but isn't always.

Now, let's cover the basic product categories.

Cleansers

When you think about it, cleansers are on your face for about fifteen seconds twice a day, hardly long enough to have any therapeutic effect on your skin. If you have normal to dry skin, a cleanser that doesn't dry out or strip oil off your skin is best, and a liquid cleanser, in particular, can be great for this. Contrary to popular opinion, you don't need to feel that squeaky feeling for your skin to be clean (that squeaky feeling is just the soap stripping all your natural oils off your skin). As long as the product is not overly irritating or drying, it's fine. If you have very oily skin, on the other hand, you're likely best off with a cleanser that's formulated specifically for acne or your skin type; these do tend to be drying—a good thing for some of us.

Some good cleansers for various skin types include:

- Cetaphil Gentle Skin Cleanser—for dry or sensitive skin (available at your drugstore)
- Cetaphil Daily Facial Cleanser for Normal to Oily Skin—for normal to oily skin (available at your drugstore)
- Dove Sensitive Skin Foaming Facial Cleanser—for dry or sensitive skin (available at your drugstore)

- Éminence Lemon Cleanser—an organic product for normal to dry skin (available online)
- Lancôme Galatée Confort Comforting Milky Creme Cleanser—for dry skin (available at department stores)
- Laura Mercier One-Step Cleanser—for normal to oily skin (available at department stores)
- Neutrogena Oil-Free Acne Wash Foam Cleanser—for oily or acne-prone skin (available at your drugstore)
- Md Formulations Facial Cleanser Foaming—for normal to oily skin (available at dermatologists' offices or online stores)

Sunscreens

You've heard it before, but it's really true: *Sunscreen is the most important product you can use on your skin every day.* The more damage to your skin cells from sunlight that you can prevent, the better your skin will be for years to come. If you have preteen or teenage children, particularly if you live in a sunny climate, encourage them to start using sunscreen on a daily basis on their faces.

Sunscreens and sun protection are the single best way to prevent prematurely aged skin, sunburns, leathery-looking skin, skin cancers, and the deadly skin cancer, melanoma (in fact, melanoma is the biggest cause of cancer deaths among kids in their twenties).

There are many types of skin, with different colors, textures, oiliness or dryness, and pore size. Here I'll focus on the three main skin types: oily, dry, and normal.

How to choose a sunscreen.   Choose a sunscreen based on your skin type, your climate, and the intensity of your sun exposure. For oily skin, choose a gel, powder, or very light lotion for your sunscreen. For normal skin, choose a lotion or a light cream, and for dry skin, a rich cream. All sunscreens that are creams and lotions have a moisturizing base. Many people don't need an extra moisturizer in addition to their sunscreen. For example, during the summer in Seattle, when we have about 30 percent

humidity, I don't use a separate moisturizer with my sunscreen. I have a normal skin type with a slightly oily T zone (forehead, nose, and chin). In the winter, however, when the central heating is on all season, then I use a moisturizer underneath my sunscreen.

Understanding SPFs.   Don't be fooled. The SPF indicates only UVB protection, *not* UVA. You might, for instance, be wearing an SPF 60 and, regardless of your skin type, still be at risk for skin cancer, wrinkles, and burns from UVA *if the sunscreen doesn't contain a UVA blocker.* Nor does the term "broad spectrum" on the bottle guarantee UVA protection, because even if the product contains only a minuscule amount of UVA blocker, it can still bear the label for "broad spectrum" coverage. Sunscreens that have 5 to 10 percent zinc or titanium or 3 percent Mexoryl are best.

The SPF tells you only how much longer you can be in the sun without burning. For instance, if you would normally burn in thirty minutes with no sunscreen, then an SPF 30 would allow you to be out fifteen

WHY YOU NEED TO TAKE VITAMIN D

What about Vitamin D and sunscreens? Vitamin D is made in our skin in response to sunlight on skin. Vitamin D is critical for bone strength and now, from a recent study, seems to help prevent several different types of cancer. Many of us in northern climates and those of us who use sunscreen don't get enough. Find out if you have enough with a simple blood test. Ask your doctor to add a 25-OH vitamin D test at your next appointment. You need between 600 and 1,200 IU of vitamin D3 (cholecalciferol), depending on your age and level of nutrition. If you are deficient, your doctor will prescribe more. Vitamin D3 is also found in milk—four glasses will give you most of what you need if you're not already deficient.

hours without burning. How many of us are out for fifteen hours? As long as you use an SPF 15, what really matters is the quality of the sunscreen ingredients, not the SPF. The higher-SPF sunscreens sometimes have better UVA blockers but not always.

Sunscreens for sports.   Fit your sunscreen to your sports and circumstances. For example, if you're outdoors midday in the summer, skiing at high altitude, hiking at altitude, or on vacation somewhere warm, you should layer two sunscreens on your face, neck, chest and hands—usually a chemical sunscreen with Mexoryl as a base and then a mineral-containing sunscreen with zinc and titanium. If you're swimming outdoors, try the inexpensive Coppertone Sport on your body (or wear a surfers' "rash guard" on the top half) and then use Blue Lizard Australian Sunscreen or SkinCeuticals Sport UV Defense SPF 45 with zinc (both wear like iron) on your face, neck, and chest.

This still will not eliminate all the UV damage to your skin cells. The only sunscreens that block out every single ray of damaging radiation are those white, opaque zincs that climbers wear on Mount Everest. But most of us can't wear this kind of sunscreen without looking ridiculous, so it's not very realistic!

Here are some good daily use sunscreens:

- Neutrogena Healthy Defense SPF 30 Daily Moisturizer (available at your drugstore)
- Colorescience Sunforgettable SPF 30 Brush—powder sunscreen for all skin types, but especially for oily skin (available online and at dermatologists' offices)
- La Roche-Posay Anthelios SX—SPF 15 and 60 (available online and at dermatologists' offices)
- Clinique City Block Sheer Oil-Free Daily Face Protector—SPF15—normal/oily (available at department stores)
- Lancôme UV Expert 20 with Mexoryl SX—SPF 20 (available at department stores)
- SkinMedica Environmental Defense Sunscreen SPF 30 (available online and at dermatologists' offices)

- Blue Lizard Face Sunscreen SPF 30 (available online and at drugstores)
- Cetaphil Daily Facial Moisturizer SPF 15 with Parsol 1789 (available at your drugstore)
- Colorescience My Favorite Eyes Cream Wand—doesn't list an SPF rating but has 22 percent zinc (available online and at dermatologists' offices)
- Dermalogica Total Eye Care SPF 15 (available at salons)
- Murad Essential-C Eye Cream SPF 15 (available online and at salons)

Toners

Here's where you can save some time and money. Toners are generally useless in my book. Though they're meant to remove "residues," I don't think it's a problem if a few molecules of a gentle cleanser get left behind on your skin after washing! They also supposedly restore the pH balance of your skin (your pH comes from the natural oils and sweat on your skin). But if you're using a gentle cleanser, it shouldn't much change the pH balance of your skin, because it's not removing your natural oil. What's more, studies have shown that your skin will replenish its natural pH balance in fifteen to thirty minutes after you wash it. If you love toners, it's fine to use them, but they're not really necessary.

Moisturizers

These deserve some attention because moisturizers *are* worth using. Particularly if you have dry skin, moisturizers will help to prevent fine lines and improve the appearance of your skin over time. We've all had the experience of being dry, applying a moisturizer, and having our skin instantly look better. Moisturizers work to retard your skin's natural loss of moisture as well as add moisture back in.

In general, if you have oily skin, you'll want to use a moisturizer like a gel that will hydrate (add water to) your skin but won't add more oil. If you have normal skin, use a lotion or light cream. If you are very dry, use a heavy cream that takes a minute or two to absorb into your skin and apply it more frequently than once or twice a day. *Everyone* should use a moisturizer around their eye area and on their necks because we all have very few oil glands in those areas. If you're oily through the T-zone area, just use your moisturizer on your eye area, your cheeks, and your neck.

Each of the basic types of skin is both a blessing and a curse. If you have oily skin, you have your own natural moisturizer and less tendency toward wrinkles. But you'll have more of a tendency toward acne and larger pores. If you have dry skin, you'll have a greater tendency toward wrinkles but much less tendency toward acne and large pores. There's something positive about each skin type.

Here are some good moisturizers:

- Bobbi Brown Hydrating Face Cream—for normal to dry skin (available at department stores)
- Cetaphil Moisturizing Lotion—for normal, sensitive skin (available at your drugstore)
- Cetaphil Moisturizing Cream—for dry, sensitive skin (available at your drugstore)
- Éminence Naseberry Treatment Cream—an organic product for dry skin (available online and at salons)
- Éminence Wild Plum Eye Cream (an organic product available at salons and online stores)
- Estée Lauder Clear Difference Advanced Oil-Control Hydrator—for oily and blemish-prone skin (available at department stores)
- Innovative Skincare Firming Complex—dry (available at dermatologists' offices and online stores)
- Laura Mercier Eyedration—firming eye cream (available at department store)
- Neutrogena Healthy Skin Lotion—for normal to dry skin (available at your drugstore)
- Olay Total Restoration Lotion—for normal to dry skin (available at your drugstore)

- SkinCeuticals Emollience—for normal to dry skin (available online and at dermatologists' offices)
- SkinCeuticals Hydrating B5 Gel—for oily skin (available online and at dermatologists' offices)

Repair Creams

The only products that have been proven to work to reduce wrinkles at this time are the vitamin-A cousins (Retin-A, Renova, Tazorac) some antioxidants like Vitamin C serums, some hydroxy acids, and possibly creams containing cell-growth factors or peptides. Let's discuss these.

Vitamin-A Creams

Vitamin-A creams are still the gold standard for repair of sun-damaged and aging skin. They also help to prevent precancerous lesions and skin cancer. There's nothing better available in a cream form. Everyone who can tolerate them should be using one!

The Vitamin-A creams go by all sorts of names like Renova, Retin-A, Tazorac, tretinoin (generic Renova and Retin-A), and Retin-A Micro (all available by prescription only). Retinol is a weaker form available without a prescription. But there are several Retinol products that are almost as strong as the prescription form.

Some women may experience irritation when using a vitamin-A cream, but if you have problems, first try washing with a gentle cleanser, applying a light moisturizer and then letting your skin rest for ten to fifteen minutes; then, use a pea-sized amount for your entire face. Renova is the best for dry or over-forty skin because it has a moisturizing base. Apply these products at night because light inactivates them. You *must* use a daily sunscreen if you're using Vitamin-A creams.

What Are Antioxidants?

It seems as if almost every skin-care product now has an added "antioxidant," and many women want to know if they really work. An antioxidant is any substance that slows or stops free-radical damage to cells. What is

GOOD DAILY SKIN CARE: A SAMPLE ROUTINE

For a good daily routine, you don't need to spend a lot nor make it too complicated. Here's a basic list of what you'll need to do:

AM

Wash with a gentle cleanser.
Apply "repair," like an antioxidant or moisturizer.
Apply sunscreen—don't forget the neck, chest, backs of hands.
Apply eye sunscreen.

PM

Wash with a gentle cleanser.
Apply moisturizer—wait ten minutes (this step and the following can be reversed).
Apply prescription Renova or another "repair" cream.
Apply eye cream.

If you have very oily or acne-prone skin, it's fine to omit or limit the moisturizing step. And, if you're using prescription skin creams, put those on after washing and before the other steps unless told otherwise by your doctor. Exfoliate gently once or twice a week.

free-radical damage to cells? When natural light damages skin cells, extra electrons (now we're talking molecules) start floating around looking for a home. When those extra electrons find a home (often a cell), they usually damage those cells when latching on. This then triggers inflammation and cell injury. Anything that slows down the injury process is referred to as an "antioxidant."

Antioxidants in Skin Creams

Many vitamins, such as Vitamins A, C, and E have antioxidant properties. Coenzymes, such as alpha-lipoic acid and coenzyme Q10, also contain antioxidants, as do many plant-derived compounds. Not surprisingly, more and more creams and cosmetics feature these antioxidants. In fact, there is good evidence to suggest that some antioxidants, like vitamins C and E *in a serum form,* have significant preventive and repairing effects for sun damage. Specifically, we know that Vitamin C serums lasts about twenty-four hours on the skin. But while we think antioxidants may help to reduce the damage to skin cells by natural light, a number of questions remain.

For instance, does sun exposure or air pollution change the amount of time that antioxidants last on our skin? How much is needed of these different antioxidants? What happens when they're combined (as they often are), and do they even get to where they would help (the skin is a good barrier)? Since free-radical damage to the skin is constant and extensive, how much antioxidant is needed to stop it? Also, do internal antioxidants taken in pill form help skin in the same way and, if so, in what doses? Unfortunately, we really don't have any idea at this point.

Still, even with these questions, it's a good idea to use a repair cream that contains antioxidants or cell growth factors, including one of the following:

- Prescription Renova/Retin-A/tretinoin—vitamin-A cream (ask your doctor)
- SkinMedica Retinol Complex—with vitamin-A cousin Retinol (available online and at dermatologists' offices)
- SkinCeuticals C E Ferulic—with three antioxidants (available at dermatologists' offices)
- Neutrogena Healthy Skin Anti-Wrinkle Cream—with Retinol, for dry to normal skin (available at your drugstore)
- Lancôme Paris Régenerie Crème—with Retinol (available at department stores)
- TNS Recovery Complex—with cellular growth extracts (available at dermatologists' offices and online stores)
- Replenix Cream—with antioxidant green tea with 90 percent polyphenol isolates (available online and at dermatologists' offices)

- Olay Regenerist—with antioxidants (available at your drugstore)
- Éminence Eight Greens Youth Serum (available online and at salons)
- Allergan Prevage MD—with antioxidant idebenone (available online and at dermatologists' offices)
- Neutrogena Visibly Firm Eyecream, Active Copper Formula (available at your drugstore)
- Replenix Intensive Eye Lightening Serum—with peptides and vitamin K (available online and at dermatologists' offices)
- SkinCeuticals Eye Balm—with soy (available online and at dermatologists' offices)
- SkinWithin EyeBright—with peptides (available online and at salons)

HOW TO PREVENT AND TREAT IRRITATION FROM PRODUCTS

Almost everyone can use one of the antioxidants or vitamin-A creams without getting irritated by following these instructions, even if you've had trouble in the past. If you *don't* get irritated easily it's fine to use the Renova, Tazorac, or vitamin C first, under your moisturizer. If you follow these instructions and are still having problems, see your dermatologist.

- Use a gentle cleanser that doesn't strip oil off your skin. Pat your skin dry after cleansing and apply your moisturizer, then *wait ten to twenty minutes* until your skin is completely dry but well moisturized.
- Take a pea-sized (and I mean pea-sized) amount of the cream or serum and dot it all over your face, rubbing in the tiny amount—avoid the eyelids.
- If you're very dry, wait another ten to fifteen minutes and apply even more moisturizer over the vitamin-A cream.
- Always apply your vitamin-A cream at night—it's inactivated by light.

- If you're still irritated, even with the above, then try using it every other night instead of every night.
- If you're *still* irritated, try diluting it half and half with your moisturizer before applying it.
- Always use a UVA/UVB blocking sunscreen every morning.

CONSUMER REPORTS WEIGHS IN

In a recent *Consumer Reports* study, entitled "Wrinkle Creams: Selling Hope in a Jar," nine top-selling wrinkle creams were tested for twelve weeks on women between ages thirty and seventy with lighter skin (the skin type most susceptible to fine lines and wrinkles). Each cream was tested by seventeen to twenty-three women, and each woman used the test product on one side of her face and the lab's standard moisturizer on the other for comparison. The women did not know which was which. The researchers then examined the women's skin using a high-tech optical device that detects changes as little as one-six-thousandth of an inch in wrinkle depth and skin roughness in the crow's foot area. The lab technicians evaluated each woman in person and took more than a thousand photographs.

Will it surprise you to learn that the researchers did not find any improvement that was visible to the naked eye? Their measuring devices were so precise, however, that they did discover some very slight improvement for a few products on some women, but the improvement could not be detected by the human eye. Nor was there any correlation between price and effectiveness, something I think we women already know!

Interestingly, their research did reveal that every product performed slightly better in some women but failed completely in others, confirming that skin is alive, metabolically active, with its own unique requirements and responses.

Of nine products that they tested, Olay Regenerist (the lotion, cream, and serum) was the most effective by a small margin. It was also one of the less costly that they tested, so that was their recommendation.

Lancôme Paris Régenerie and RoC Retin-Ox were also found to be slightly more effective in combating wrinkles. Of average effectiveness were Neutrogena Visibly Firm night cream with Active Copper, Avon Anew Alternative Intensive Age Treatment, L'Oréal Paris Dermo-Expertise, and StriVectin-SD Intensive Concentrate for Stretch Marks.

The article concluded by pointing out the fact that if you want dramatic visible changes to your skin, "You are probably going to need products available only from your doctor—and even then, don't expect miracles." They recommended retinoids, or the vitamin-A derivatives already discussed, including Renova, Retin-A, and Tazorac. They also pointed out that hydroxyl-acid peels, which we'll discuss in the next chapter, done in a series, are also effective in stimulating collagen and reversing sun damage.

SIX MYTHS ABOUT PRODUCTS

I think every one of us will see ourselves when we read this list, including me. I have definitely fallen into some of these traps—some of them more than once.

1. Products have to cost a lot to be good. There are some excellent drugstore products made by large international cosmetic companies that cost between ten and twenty-five dollars. You don't have to spend four hundred dollars on a serum to get good skin care.
2. The newest, latest, greatest thing is better. Usually the only advantage to the newest, latest, greatest thing is its marketing muscle. Some of the best products on the market are tried and true with long track records of success. For example, vitamin-A cousins (like Renova and Retinol) have been shown over many years to help prevent skin cancers, normalize sun-damaged cells, and prevent wrinkles.

3. Creams can really make us look significantly younger. There is, at this writing, absolutely no cream on the market that will make you look five years younger just by using the cream. Darn! The fact is, the only products that have been proven over time to improve skin are sunscreens, vitamin-A cousins (like Renova and Retinol), vitamin-C serums (not creams), a few other antioxidants, and hydroxy acids.

4. Cosmetic companies spend a lot of money on research. Some do and some don't. It depends on what you mean by "research." If you mean researching how to market and sell it, yes. And cosmetic companies do spend time and money trying to figure out how to put the latest "discovery," like green tea, into a topical cream or lotion. But take note that these companies almost never do the type of research that is standard in any scientific laboratory, like controlled trials comparing the new product with older products that we know work well. Just because a product sounds exotic or rare does not mean it has any benefit for skin whatsoever in a cream form.

5. If something is good for me to eat or drink, it must be good in a cream. Absolutely untrue. Even many tablet supplements have not been shown to be beneficial to skin in the long run. And, even if something is beneficial to take in a tablet form, putting it in a cream changes the way it reacts with cells. The skin is such a good barrier layer that it's very difficult to get active ingredients through the barrier layer into the part of the skin where it might actually do some good. What's more, the companies that put supplements into cream don't spend much time or money on the research *in actual patients* to show if it works or not.

6. Plant-based creams are always safe. Any dermatologist will tell you that we have all seen many, many allergic reactions to creams, lotions, gels, and ointments. Some of these are due to plant ingredients. Think about all the people who have allergies to plants and imagine what happens when similar plants get put on their skin in a cream form.

HOW TO THINK ABOUT THE PRODUCTS YOU BUY

To recap, here are the types of products that have been proven over the years with good science to help your skin:

- gentle cleansers
- moisturizers
- sunscreens
- repair creams with vitamin-A cousins (like Renova and Retinol), vitamin-C serums (not creams), a few other antioxidants, and hydroxy acids.

You're smart to find good products from these categories that work for your skin. That is money well spent.

All the other stuff out there on the market? Go ahead and play with it—have fun! Talk to your friends about it. Make it a luxury for yourself that is part of your own self-care. Go ahead and dream that you may find the fountain of youth. But don't mislead yourself into thinking that your hard-earned cash can get you the facelift in a bottle. And do try only one new product at time. That way you'll know what causes a reaction if you get one. Even if it is the algae cream that cost you $150!

THE BOTTOM LINE

- Keep it simple. The women with the best skin I've ever seen for their ages have fairly simple daily routines.
- Use sunscreen on your face, neck, and chest every day. Don't forget to make sure you are getting 400 to 800 units or more of vitamin D per day and plenty of calcium so your bones stay strong.
- Beware of the latest antioxidant madness, which consists of throwing a gazillion antioxidants randomly into skin care creams.
- If you have allergic or sensitive skin, try the Free & Clear product line that also goes by the name of Vanicream. It's free of all plant extracts and of many of the preservatives, lanolin, fragrances, and

such that can irritate people with very sensitive skin (see *www.psico.com*).

- For more advice on products go to *surgeryfreemakeover.com*.
- The looks of your skin and the health of your skin are very closely correlated. Healthy skin is usually beautiful skin. But don't get caught in the beauty trap. Our skin doesn't have to be perfect. There's a happy balance for all of us.

2

BEYOND THE CREAMS

YOUR QUICK GUIDE TO BOTOX, FILLERS, LASERS, AND OTHER COSMETIC TREATMENTS

The life of the modern woman is *busy*. Between working, getting kids to all their school and extracurricular events, figuring out healthy meals (or just *some* meal), volunteering (women make up the backbone of the volunteer force in every city), trying to stay in shape, and getting a great haircut, it's all most of us can do to stay afloat. You might just be looking for a very quick overview of skin-care options right now to see if they make sense for you and your lifestyle. After reading chapter 1 on products, you already know that the daily product workhorses are a gentle cleanser; your daily sunscreen; moisturizers to keep your skin hydrated; an eye cream, including one for morning with sunscreen in it; and repair creams and serums like the vitamin-A cousins, vitamin-C serums, hydroxy-acid creams, and possibly creams with antioxidants, peptides, and cell-growth factors.

But what if you need more than products? By the time most of my patients over forty come to me, they've more or less realized that a magical cream won't give them the makeover they'd like. They know they've got to take more initiative to repair some of the damage to their skin, but many don't want to do something as drastic as go under the knife for plastic surgery. So, what other options or procedures are available to them? This chapter gives you an overview of some of the surgery-free techniques that can be quite effective in eliminating wrinkles, smoothing skin, and addressing other concerns of forty-plus skin. These treatments will all be discussed in much more detail later in the book. But this overview will introduce you to them and also give you a handy place to refer back to.

Here are the most frequent cosmetic antiaging treatments. There are many others discussed in this book, but these are the most common:

- Botox Cosmetic
- wrinkle and lip fillers like Restylane and Juvederm
- lasers for redness and blotchiness, brown spots, or age spots
- lasers like the Fraxel for wrinkles, brown spots and texture problems
- lasers for hair removal
- radiofrequency like Thermage and Titan for skin tightening
- peels and microdermabrasion

BOTOX

Botox is a clear, injectable liquid, tiny amounts of which relax overactive facial muscles. Its benefits include relaxing frown lines, relaxing horizontal forehead lines, lifting the eyebrows a little, relaxing smile lines around the eye (crow's feet), relaxing upper-lip lines, relaxing the muscle that causes chin dimpling, helping to fix a smile that shows too much gum on the upper teeth, and other uses. It is FDA-approved for frown lines and is used "off-label" for other areas of the face.

Ironically, Botox is one of the safest procedures around today, even though it initially may sound the scariest. Botox has been used since the mid-1980s and has an outstanding safety profile (though it's not used during pregnancy because no research has been done). It was first used to give relief to medical patients who had uncontrollable twitching or muscle spasms, often in the eye area.

When you get Botox, tiny amounts of the botulinum toxin are injected directly into the muscle that is overactive. But rest assured, when injected correctly the toxin doesn't travel anywhere else in the body; it stays in the muscle, binding to the receptor between the nerve and muscle. This allows the muscle to stop contracting, relaxes the muscle, and provides a smoother look. The results are temporary, but as time goes on, the results last longer and longer.

Cost and longevity.   How much Botox will you need? This depends on your face and how many areas you're treating. Men's faces have larger muscles, so they almost always need more than women. Many of my patients need less Botox as time goes on because muscles become less active. Expect to pay approximately four hundred to one thousand dollars per treatment, depending on how many areas you are treating, your age, and the size of your facial muscles. Botox needs to be repeated every three to six months, depending on your particular face and issues. Most of my patients come two to three times a year, but expect three to four treatments during the first year.

THE LINE FILLERS—JUVEDERM, RESTYLANE, AND COSMOPLAST

Fillers like Restylane and Juvederm are natural sugars that are injected into lines, creases, and grooves in your face. They give a near-instantaneous lifting and filling of medium to deep wrinkles. They're also injected into the lips to provide plumping or more volume or definition to the lips.

CosmoPlast and CosmoDerm are second-generation collagens, meaning they're made from a human-cell line grown in the lab; the same cells are grown over and over again so there's no change in the DNA. These are best for defining the border of the lips and filling tiny upper-lip lines and small lines or acne scars elsewhere on the face. They don't require allergy testing like the first-generation collagens (Zyplast and Zyderm), because CosmoPlast and CosmoDerm aren't made from an animal source.

Cost and longevity.   Restylane and Juvederm will generally last four to nine months, depending on how much product is used and how it's layered into your the skin; most patients need one to two syringes per appointment. Expect to pay four hundred to seven hundred dollars per syringe. CosmoDerm usually lasts two to four months and Cosmo-Plast three to five months, depending on the area injected. Once again, expect to pay four hundred to seven hundred dollars per syringe.

Below is a quick cheat sheet for what each filler is made of.

Restylane/Perlane	Hyaluronic acid (HA)—made in Sweden—no human or animal DNA (No HOADNA)
Juvederm/Juvederm Ultra Plus	HA made in France (NO HOADNA)
Sculptra	A type of lactic acid—Poly-L-Lactic Acid—made in Italy owned by French company Sanofi-Aventis(NO HOADNA)
Hyalaform	An HA made from rooster combs
CosmoPlast/CosmoDerm— collagen	Human collagen made from one cell line in the lab so it has a good safety profile
Isolagen—collagen made from you—need a piece of own skin	There were lab problems several years ago but seem to have been solved. Expensive.
Radiesse—calcium hydroxylapatite	Similar to bone and cartilage—has been associated with problems in and around the lips

* I use some of these products in my medical practice, but I have no financial ties of any kind to these products.

Risks.   Juvederm, Restylane, CosmoDerm, and CosmoPlast are quite safe, with most of the risks being temporary bruising, swelling, or redness where the filler is injected. There are rare risks like scarring, so be sure you have a competent injector and read your consent forms. Other fillers have more risks and are discussed later in the book.

SCULPTRA

Sculptra (the generic name is poly-L-lactic acid, or PLA) is a form of synthetic lactic acid. You may know lactic acid as the natural substance that our muscles produce after exercise. Polylactic acid is simply lactic-acid molecules stuck together in a chain. Sculptra contains no animal products and no human DNA. It works to stimulate the body's own cells to make more collagen, which is why its effects are so long lasting. Sculptra gradually disappears by the action of the body's own enzymes. To minimize discomfort during injection, Sculptra is mixed with lidocaine, a local anesthetic.

While Sculptra has full approval in the European union and Canada, it has limited FDA approval (HIV only—other uses are "off-label") in the United States Full approval is expected in 2008.

Maintenance and costs.   Sculptra lasts approximately two years once the series of treatments is completed, but I would also recommend one maintenance treatment a year to maintain a consistent look. Costs are about nine hundred to thirteen hundred dollars per vial.

Risks.   There are more risks with Sculptra than with Juvederm or Restylane, the hyaluronic-acid fillers. See chapter 6 for details.

LASER TREATMENTS

Cosmetic laser treatments can be excellent for the following:

· redness and dilated blood vessels on the face or legs
· blotchiness, brown spots, and age spots

- most types of wrinkles
- hair removal

Lasers are simple in a way because they are just light that's focused into a powerful single beam to target problems in your skin, such as too much pigment or blotchiness, too many blood vessels or wrinkles, or too much hair. An IPL (intense pulsed light) is just a laser cousin that blends different wavelengths to achieve its result—it's like a blended wine instead of a wine made from just one type of grape.

What's confusing to most women is that there seem to be so many different types of lasers. Approximately twenty different companies make more than a hundred different lasers. But few have really stood the test of time, and those are the ones discussed in this book.

Cost and longevity. This depends on what laser treatment is being done and how large an area of skin is being treated. Treating a few hairs on your chin is much less expensive than a man's entire hairy back! Remember, there's an initial repair phase followed by a maintenance phase.

For repair of redness and vessels, expect usually a series of three to five treatments followed by a treatment once or twice a year for maintenance. A full-face treatment is generally four hundred to six hundred dollars in a reputable doctor's office. The lasers and IPLs used in salons are not as powerful as the ones used in doctors' offices.

For repair of brown spots, expect usually a series of three to five treatments followed by one or two treatments a year for maintenance. A full-face treatment is generally four hundred to six hundred dollars in a reputable doctor's office.

Wrinkles and acne scars are typically treated with fractional or conventional resurfacing lasers. For repair, expect a series of three to five treatments (except for a carbon dioxide or erbium laser, in which case one is enough). Maintenance depends on the type of laser. Costs vary from one thousand to five thousand (carbon dioxide laser) for a full face treatment.

For unwanted hair, unless you have hormone abnormalities, a series of four to six treatments followed by maintenance one to three times a year is average. Costs vary widely by area but for the underarm area an initial package would range from four hundred to nine hundred dollars.

Risks.   In expert hands, the risks of a laser treatment are very small: usually a little swelling and/or an increase in redness or the brown spots for three to seven days after the treatment. A good laser center will prepare you for those. But there are big risks with lasers in general—severe burns, permanent scarring, permanent discoloration, and even death are possible in untrained, inexperienced, or unethical hands. Stay away from medi-spas and mall clinics unless they have a full-time dermatologist on site.

SKIN TIGHTENING: THERMAGE AND TITAN

Thermage is a radiofrequency (soundwave) skin-tightening system that has become more popular in the past five years. It is used primarily on the face, eyelids, and neck. Thermage helps to prevent further sagging and reduces the inevitable sagging that we all notice on our eyelids, around our cheeks and midface, and particularly along our jawlines. Thermage can deliver significant but not dramatic tightening for many patients. It's *not* a substitute for a facelift for jowls or a significantly sagging neck. The tightening occurs over six months following the treatment, so the effect is gradual rather than immediate.

Titan is an infrared laser that produces similar results to the Thermage. Its original incarnation was not very effective, but it, too, has evolved and is more effective now. Its main disadvantage compared to Thermage is that it takes three or four treatments to get the same effect as one Thermage—and it's more painful. The costs are approximately equal. One Titan treatment is less, but remember, you'll need a series of treatments.

Maintenance and costs.   The tightening from a Thermage treatment lasts one to two years. For my patients in their thirties and forties, every other year seems like a reasonable interval given the data on tightening. As you get into your fifties, sixties, and seventies, perhaps you'll want to try yearly treatments at that point. Thermage is also very helpful for maintaining facelifts. A full-face Thermage can range from twenty-two hundred to over three thousand dollars.

Risks.   The real risk with Thermage is that you might not respond. About 5 to 10 percent of patients don't see any visible tightening with Thermage, but even then it helps to prevent more sagging. There were some indentations reported with the first generation of Thermage tips (the part that touches the face), but the tips and protocol were revised—and no similar problems have been reported in several years. Occasionally, small, superficial burns can occur.

PEELS AND MICRODERMABRASION

Both light peels and microdermabrasion are good ways to refresh dull skin (think glow), unclog pores, and help with milder forms of acne and melasma. They are performed usually by aestheticians in a dermatologist's office or at salons.

Microdermabrasion is usually done either with a diamond-tipped system or a crystal-based system that vacuums crystals across your skin. The treatment is not painful at all, and you emerge with skin that appears more youthful and smooth. Medical offices usually offer a higher level of training and can purchase medical-grade devices that may not be available to salons or spas.

Light peels are generally alpha- or beta-hydroxy acid based and have a similar effect to microdermabrasion. They help slough off the outer dead layer of skin, increase the cell turnover rate, which makes the texture of the skin slightly better, giving it a fresher and more youthful appearance. They also unclog pores. Light peels are generally done by aestheticians in a doctor's office or at a salon. Medium peels are roughly defined as peels that cause peeling anywhere from five to ten days with mild to

TREATMENT	COST RANGE
Botox	
Frown lines	$300–500
Frown lines, forehead, crows' feet	$500–1,000 or more
Restylane/Juvederm	
Fill grooves from nose to mouth	$400–700 per syringe
Plump the lips	$400–700 per syringe
CosmoPlast	
Lip lines	$400–700 per syringe
Sculptra	
Filling in hollow cheeks	$1,000–1,900 per treatment
Filling in under the eyes	$400–800 per treatment
Laser	
Photorejuvenation (IPL): Face and Chest	$1,500–3,000 face—series of five
Fractional Laser	
Full face	$1,000–1,500 per treatment
Thermage	
Full face	$2,200–3,200
Peels & Microdermabrasion	$75–200 per treatment

moderate pinkness or redness. These are generally performed by a nurse or a doctor. Lasers have replaced deep phenol peels completely.

Costs and maintenance.   Both microdermabrasion and light peels take anywhere from thirty minutes to an hour and cost anywhere from seventy to two hundred dollars per treatment depending on what's being done. Most clinics or salons offer a package discount for a series of treatments. After an initial series of three to five treatments, maintenance could be as much as once a year (to refresh mild sun damage after summer) to monthly (for active acne).

Risks.   With light peels or microdermabrasion some temporary discoloration could occur for two to eight weeks. Temporary pinkness and sun sensitivity for a week or two is another possible side effect. Abrasions or blisters are rare.

THE BOTTOM LINE

- Your daily care is the most important thing you can do to for your skin, but it probably won't be enough if you're over forty or have significant sun damage.
- When considering Botox, fillers, lasers, and Thermage, be careful to go to only a *board-certified* dermatologist or a plastic surgeon's office. Light peels or microdermabrasion are fine at good salons. A treatment won't seem like a "deal" if you end up with a complication.

PART TWO
YOUR PERSONAL SKIN CONSULTATION

3

YOUR FOREHEAD

I'm tired of all this nonsense about beauty being only skin-deep.
That's deep enough. What do you want, an adorable pancreas?
—Jean Kerr

Several years ago, a school principal came into my office. She was a little shy, but after a bit she confessed that what was really bothering her was that the kids at her school kept asking, "Are you mad at me?" "Did I do something?" when she felt totally fine. She finally realized that her involuntary frown lines were causing the misunderstandings! This is the perfect use for Botox in the forehead frown lines. She still comes in twice a year.

The forehead, though, should be expressive. To have it not move at all looks more than odd, in my opinion. Good Botox should allow some natural movement of the forehead so it doesn't look frozen.

If you were a fly on the wall of my exam room, you would hear comments like these:

- "I hate these frown lines because people think I'm angry when I'm not."
- "My mother has these lines, and now they've turned into ravines."
- "I always look tense and worried with these lines."
- "My forehead and eyelids feel heavy."

I've asked thousands of my patients over the years this question: Did your father or mother have frown lines like this? They almost invariably say yes. They often go on to tell me about their siblings who also have lines in exactly the same areas. Look at your parents' foreheads! Here's an opportunity to take evasive action if you don't like what you see.

Happily, most forehead problems are correctable without surgery. For many women, the first area they'd like to change on their face when they map out their surgery-free makeover is their forehead. Take a minute to ask yourself what's really bothering you about your forehead area. Some self-knowledge will save you time, money, and frustration in the long run.

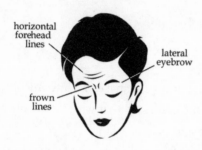

horizontal
forehead
lines

lateral
eyebrow

frown
lines

GET SPECIFIC

Make a list of your complaints before talking to your doctor about treatment options. Add anything else that you'd like to improve to feel more beautiful and confident.

- My forehead makes me look tense.
- I have permanent frown lines.
- I have lumps and bumps that don't go away on my forehead.
- I have horizontal forehead creases.
- My eyebrows are dropping.
- I look gaunt and hollow at the temples.

FIXING YOUR FROWN LINES

Problem: My frown lines have become permanent.

Best Solutions: Botox, Restylane

Frown lines are one of the easiest problems to correct for most women. It's amazing to me how many patients from all different walks of life—including moms, teachers, principals, DJs, lawyers, doctors, corporate executives, travel agents, and more—who feel completely transformed by having their brow look more relaxed, their frown lines gone.

When people look at you, the first thing they see is your eyes. If you can get rid of those vertical frown lines between your eyes, your whole demeanor will appear more relaxed. I personally use Botox in this area, and I can be exhausted and still look moderately rested. It's a minor miracle!

Restylane and Juvederm

While Botox relaxes the muscle that is contracting too much, fillers like Restylane and Juvederm *fill in* the wrinkle from underneath. They work best together if your lines are fairly deep. Using Botox *plus* a filler has longer-lasting results, but the cost is more. If you're on a budget, I'd recommend starting with Botox and then see where you are in nine months. Often, frown lines will relax enough with just Botox so that you won't need the filler and the additional expense.

Botox

Botox basics. Botox is made by Allergan, a company with a twenty-year history of making this product safely. Botox is a clear liquid that's injected with a tiny needle into overactive facial muscles to relax them; when injected into a small muscle, it doesn't travel anywhere else in the body. It gradually wears off naturally. There is also another product, Reloxin (known in other countries as Dysport), which is just coming to the American market after extensive use in Europe. It's not known yet exactly how it will compare here.

The best Botox. With Botox, there is the great, the good, the bad, and the ugly. Great Botox is customized to your individual face, taking into account factors such as which facial muscles you use the most, your facial muscle balance from side to side, your job, your social life, and the look you want (for example, natural or high glam). Great Botox requires excellent and steady injecting hands, the eye of an artist, and the passion to care about it. Great Botox injectors can be hard to find.

Good Botox is where you get the standard four or five shots into your frown lines and you go on your way. It works perfectly well, but there's not much customization. And the range of looks that these injectors can accomplish is limited. But if you have only some frown lines, good Botox can work just fine for you.

Bad Botox is everywhere. You've seen it on television: it's that completely unnatural frozen look, or worse, where the poor person almost looks like she's had a stroke, one side of her face completely different from the other. The point is, Botox is not a cookie-cutter procedure. In the hands of a good injector, it can create a marvelously natural look that makes you more refreshed- and relaxed-looking without freezing your whole forehead.

The goal of Botox is no wrinkles, not no movement!

Finding a great doctor or nurse.   First, look at your friends and ask them for recommendations. If you like the way your friend looks, chances are you'll like her doctor! Next, schedule a consultation if you can, and find out how many years the doctor or nurse has been injecting Botox (at least five years is preferable). Avoid offices that advertise; offices advertise because they aren't busy enough. Good doctors are busy. And finally check on the Botox website, which features a list of excellent offices.

What can go wrong?   It's a question patients always ask, and of course you want to be aware of the risks. But with a qualified, experienced doctor or nurse injecting, these potential problems should be rare or nonexistent.

- The frozen forehead. I call it the "Oscar-Night Freeze." We've all seen this: the face absolutely doesn't move. The result looks slightly robotic, not natural in the least. In the beginning, when working with frown lines, the corrugator muscle (the muscle that operates when people frown) may need to be completely relaxed, for a while. Once the frown line dissipates, though, it makes sense to adjust the Botox dose to allow for a little movement so that the expression looks natural. Remember, the goal is no *wrinkles,* not no *movement.*

- One or both eyebrows pop up too much. With bad Botox, one or both eyebrows are elevated so much that the arch or the last third of the eyebrow sits up too high, giving the patient a chronically surprised look. In addition, odd wrinkles can occur over the lateral brow. A good injector will know how to prevent this and how to fix it quickly (it should be no charge) with a few strategically placed drops, if it happens.

- Eyelid drooping. This is the complication you read about most often, though it's actually one of the rarest. Most of the time, the *eyebrow* has dropped, and it makes the eyelid feel heavy. If your eyelid is truly drooping after your Botox treatment, call your doctor. There are prescription drops that will temporarily help elevate the eyelid, making this problem bearable until the effects of the Botox are gone.

- "My brow feels like an elephant sat on it." This is the result of over-Botoxing the forehead, specifically the frontalis muscle, which goes all the way across the forehead and is used to raise the eyebrows. This relaxes the forehead too much, which results in a heavy feeling. When the forehead comes down, so do the eyebrows. Since some of us raise our eyebrows a lot to make the eyes feel more open when there is excess eyelid skin (called hooding), then dropping the eyebrows makes the eyelids look worse—or more hooded. If the doctor doesn't correctly perceive how much the patient uses this muscle, then too much Botox will make the eyelids and forehead feel heavy and more closed.

- Hospital stays and bootleg Botox. There have been several legal cases where doctors bought bootleg or illegal Botox. This is Botox that's used primarily for research purposes with animals. This type of Botox comes very concentrated, and the doctors involved in these cases tried to dilute it themselves. In one case in Florida, a doctor diluted it incorrectly and landed himself, his girlfriend, and a patient—the doctor injected all three of them—in the hospital for months. In another case, a doctor was diluting Botox and then putting it into Allergan Botox vials. The best way to protect yourself is to make sure your doctor has a long and excellent reputation in your community. And don't go for cheap "Botox specials"—it's often cheap for a reason! Never be injected outside a doctor's office or a medical setting. Remember those "Botox parties" held in hotels? Not a good idea.

REAL-WORLD ADVICE

Is it possible to become resistant to Botox?   Let's put it this way: It is extremely rare. If you had botulinum poisoning as a child, say, from some home-canned vegetables, you could have antibodies to it and be resistant. Also remember that Botox is used in much greater quantities for many different medical conditions with resistance only rarely, sometimes in doses that are a hundred times higher than the ones used for cosmetic purposes. We use very tiny amounts of Botox for cosmetic uses. If you suspect that you're resistant, it's far more likely that the Botox is not being injected correctly or that it's being overdiluted.

What about all these "better than Botox" cosmeceutical remedies I keep reading about, like StriVectin and Frown Ease?   For frown lines, none of the creams or patches that have claimed to be as good or better than Botox has ever worked for longer than a few hours or, at most, a few days. StriVectin published a "study" comparing itself to Botox in which one group of patients slathered the cream on their frown lines and the other group had Botox injected. The patients were then asked which group looked better—the StriVectin side or the Botox side. All of them testified the StriVectin side looked better. However, Botox takes *five days* to work after it's injected! So a comparison immediately after the injection is absurd. In addition, StriVectin is also a moisturizer, so it can make your skin look smoother immediately after being applied. This is the kind of snake-oil medicine that wastes your time and money.

What about cutting the nerves in the forehead? Doesn't this work as well as or better than Botox?   This does work, but it's awfully invasive, since it's a surgery. You would never have any movement in the area again, and to my mind it looks very unnatural. With Botox injected correctly, once you reach the maintenance phase (usually after a year or so), then some movement can be left in the forehead, resulting in a more natural look without undue wrinkling.

What's the difference between Botox and Reloxin or Dysport?   Dysport is another form of botulinum toxin that doctors have used in Europe for many years. The FDA recently approved its use in the United States. Sold under the trade name Reloxin, it's distributed by Medicis, a reputable company. Interestingly, it's the first real competition for Allergan's Botox. Almost every year, I go to Paris for the International Master Course on Aging Skin (IMCAS), and Dysport has been talked about for a number of years there. After a review of the data and talking to European physicians, I'd surmise that the only difference seems to be that Dysport may not last quite as long as Botox and may be more painful to inject. It remains to be seen if Reloxin will be a worthy opponent of Botox or not. Botox is so safe and effective; it has set the bar quite high.

My husband went in for Botox, and it cost him twice as much as it does me. Did he get ripped off?   No, probably not. Men generally need about twice as much Botox as women to get the same effect. This is because the muscles in their face are larger.

I am an African-American woman and wonder if it's safe for me to use Botox.   Yes, absolutely safe. It is safe for all ethnicities and all skin types, so you can feel comfortable going in that direction if you'd like.

I've gone twice to the same office and had Botox injections, and it doesn't seem to be working very well. What could be wrong?   It could be a couple of different things. It may be that your nurse or doctor is diluting the Botox beyond what Allergan recommends. I would find another reputable office and try a different doctor. It could also be that the Botox isn't being injected in quite the right places for your muscles. The doctor or nurse injecting should look at the way your muscles are moving before they start injecting. It may also be that you're not getting enough Botox for the size of your muscles. With very deep frown lines, it can take a year or more with Botox alone to get the area looking more relaxed. If that's the case, you might want to ask your nurse or doctor to inject a little Restylane in the area at the same time, which will give you more immediate relief from the frown lines.

HORIZONTAL FOREHEAD LINES

Problem: I have one or more horizontal lines that go across my forehead.
Best Solution: Botox

Treatment for horizontal forehead lines really depends on the depth of the lines and your age. I once had a patient, around thirty-five, who complained about her forehead lines. I looked and looked, but I couldn't see anything. After talking with her for a while, I realized that what was bothering her was the fact that her forehead moved when she talked. A friend of hers had told her about having Botox injected in her forehead lines, and my patient wanted the same for hers. I talked that patient *out* of Botox because she really had *no* wrinkles there—not even one. Even children have temporary crinkles in their foreheads when they raise their eyebrows!

For others with horizontal forehead lines while at rest, Botox works quite well. Unlike with frown lines, where I treat both men and women equally aggressively, I treat horizontal forehead lines more aggressively in women. I think women look natural with a smooth forehead, as long as the forehead moves some with facial expressions and doesn't feel too heavy. A light touch is the key.

With men, particularly men over forty, I think they look unnatural without any horizontal forehead lines at all. I do use Botox in horizontal forehead lines in my male patients, but my goal is to diminish or soften the lines rather than eliminate them.

Can forehead lines be prevented by starting Botox early?   There is some disagreement among experts in the field about how much Botox should be used to prevent problems before they develop. To my mind, why spend money on trying to prevent a problem that may never develop in the first place? Not everyone develops forehead lines that are notice-able, just as not everyone develops frown lines. If lines do appear and bother you, you can begin treatment then. It's true that if you wait for treatment for years and the lines are very deep—more crevasses than lines—they may not ever go away completely. My recommendation would be to start treating the problem when it first occurs so that it re-solves completely. Regardless, I discourage patients who are under the age of thirty from starting Botox for forehead lines, unless there really is something there to treat.

I had Botox done and my forehead felt so heavy that I couldn't stand it. The feeling lasted for two or three weeks. Does this mean I can't use Botox?   This is probably due to one of two problems. Either too much Botox was injected for the size and activity of your forehead muscles, or you're using your forehead muscles to lift your eyebrows because you have upper-eyelid hooding. When your forehead relaxed, your eyebrows dropped, and that's the heaviness you feel. Sometimes it's a little bit of both. If it's the latter, you may need to surgically remove the excess skin on the upper eyelid before using Botox again on the horizontal lines— you can still treat your frown lines.

I am an actor, and while my forehead lines are making me look older, I need to be able to show emotions by wrinkling my forehead. Can I use

Botox under the circumstances?   Yes, but definitely go to an expert. I've worked with actors who want to retain movement in their faces, and for them I do what I call my "microdroplet" Botox injections. With care, it is possible to inject very small amounts to soften the lines but not eliminate too much movement.

FOREHEAD LIFTS—THE REAL STORY

Problem: My eyebrows are sagging, especially at the outer edges.

Best Solutions: Nonsurgical forehead lift with Thermage or plastic surgery

When someone says forehead lift, most of us think of plastic surgery. The older surgical method was quite invasive and involved making an incision all the way across the top of the head. These scars often didn't heal well, sometimes getting infected, which caused widening of the scars or even areas that refused to heal. Some patients experienced hair loss around the scar area, and others ended up with that chronically surprised look because their eyebrows were positioned too high.

Now, surgical forehead lifts are mostly done with an endoscope (a small scope that helps the surgeon visualize the area without having to make such a large incision). This results in two smaller scars in the hairline that are not as problematic as the older, large scars.

Even with the new procedure, though, there is the risk of that chronically surprised look, and the results from the new procedure do not seem to last as long. Many patients have told me that two or three years later, they don't really see much difference from the original problem. Surgical forehead lifts can also demand a two-week recovery period, and the cost of the procedure—in the range of three thousand to ten thousand dollars—is prohibitive for many patients.

Thankfully, there is a nonsurgical forehead lift option done with Thermage, a soundwave-based technology (see chapter 6 for all the details on Thermage) that has been around for five years. It's most effective for patients who need only mild to moderate elevation of the eyebrows and can be repeated several times for better results. (It will not give you the same results as a surgical lift, however. If you need a lot of lift, surgery may be better.)

As discussed in chapter 2, Thermage uses a sound wave (radiofrequency) to tighten the skin. A cooled one-and-a-half-inch (about three centimeters) tip attached to a handpiece is run over the entire forehead and temple area multiple times (go to *surgeryfreemakeover.com* to see a video). This will tighten the skin above the eyebrows enough to raise the eyebrows anywhere from one to fourmillimeters. That may not sound like much, but try using your hands to raise your eyebrows. Just a little bit of elevation makes a huge difference in your expression and how "open" the entire eye area looks. Two millimeters is often plenty.

Thermage has evolved just like software. The newer Thermage tips are very comfortable. So ignore what you may have heard about discomfort; that's really a thing of the past, and no sedation is needed now. I know because I've had Thermage treatments myself, and we've treated hundreds of patients with Thermage at my clinic.

A forehead lift with Thermage is a safe, nonsurgical procedure with absolutely no down time. Because no sedation is used, no driver is required, and you can walk in and out of the procedure and go immediately back to your normal activities. Almost everyone will get some elevation of the eyebrows. The procedure can be repeated six months after the initial treatment if more lift is desired. Forehead Thermage is relatively inexpensive, costing between one thousand and twenty-five hundred dollars, depending on the area of the country. Maintenance treatments are usually done yearly or every other year.

SCRUNCH AND SQUINT LINES AT THE TOP OF THE NOSE

These scrunch and squint lines at the top of your nose are different from frown lines. The scrunch lines come from the contraction of a different muscle than the one you contract when you frown. But Botox is still the best way to fix both of these problems.

Try doing this yourself in the mirror—really scrunch and squint your face and see the lines develop on your nose when you do that. You can easily see why these get more etched in the skin as time goes on. The ones on the top of the nose are called "scrunch" lines and the ones on the side of the nose, "bunny" lines.

A little bit of Botox injected here (and it takes very little) does wonders, and if your dermatologist or nurse is treating existing frown lines it's easy to treat this area at the same time. Only a few drops will usually smooth out this area. I also sometimes put a little filler—Juvederm or Restylane—under this area to support the skin if the lines have become deeply ingrained. Plumping the skin while relaxing lines is a good combination.

YOUR EYEBROW POSITION

Problem: I feel like my eyebrows are falling.
Best Solutions: Botox, Restylane or Juvederm, Thermage forehead lift

Your eyebrows feel as if they're falling because *they are* falling. As the skin in the forehead gradually loses some elasticity and structure, the skin becomes looser and the eyebrows tend to drop down.

Treatments

Here's the good news: there's a lot that you can do nonsurgically to improve this problem. Let's go through the three possibilities: Botox, a little Restylane or Juvederm, and a Thermage forehead lift.

Botox.   My patients often think I'm nuts when I suggest putting Botox underneath the outer half of the eyebrow to give them a little bit of an eyebrow lift. They say (very understandably), how can that make the eyebrow lift? Won't it make it droop? The answer is no. There's a little muscle, right underneath the eyebrow, which acts to pull *down* the eyebrow. So the Botox relaxes it and—voilà—the eyebrow tail goes up. If you've ever had Botox, you'll understand exactly what I mean about the lifting effect. It wears off, of course, as the Botox wears off, but a few millimeters of lift can make a tremendous difference. Go to the mirror and try this yourself: if you raise your outer eyebrow up with your finger, even the slightest bit, it creates a more youthful look in the entire eye area.

Restylane or Juvederm.   I don't think it would be cost effective to a patient to open an entirely new syringe just to treat the eyebrows. But if you have chosen to have one of these fillers (full details on Restylane and Juvederm in chapter 5) done on another area and you're having trouble with your eyebrows drooping, it's possible that a little bit of Restylane just under the lateral brow will help support that area as well. Again, a millimeter or two can make a big difference.

Thermage forehead lift.   We've already talked about the effect of Thermage on forehead lines and creases. And Thermage over the entire forehead and temple area works nicely to get a little lift to the eyebrows too. A good nurse or doctor performing this procedure should be able to put more pulses over the area of the outer part of the eyebrow (typically the problem area) and get even more lifting in the area that needs it most.

I often recommend combining two or three of these compatible methods to get maximum lift without surgery. In my professional opinion,

WHEN TO RUN SCREAMING OUT THE DOOR

- if you suspect that the office may be unethical for any reason
- if the office seems dirty or disorganized
- be suspicious of franchises or chains with no real roots in the community
- if there's no physician on site to deal with possible problems, preferably a board-certified dermatologist or plastic surgeon—*ask*

because the eyebrows frame the entire face as well as the eye area, eyebrow drooping is one of the problems I recommend correcting first. Treatment here has an immediate and noticeable effect on the look of the entire face.

REAL-WORLD ADVICE

When should I give up on nonsurgical options and consider getting a forehead lift? First, do you have a lot of sagging of skin in your upper eyelids? Severe upper-eyelid hooding can be corrected only by surgery. So, if you're undertaking the surgical risks already for an upper-eyelid correction, and if your eyebrows are really drooping, then adding an endoscopic forehead lift into the mix could be a good option.

If you don't have upper-eyelid problems as well, try this. Feel where your brow bone is and gauge whether or not your eyebrows are on or near the bone. If they are, consider non-surgical options first. If your eyebrows are really way down below the bone, then you may need surgery to correct the problem. I would ask the opinion of a reputable board-certified plastic surgeon and get at least two opinions.

I had a surgical forehead lift and I ended up with that surprised look. Is there anything I can do to correct it now? Time itself will help because the skin gradually relaxes as we get older. Using Botox in the forehead to fully relax the forehead muscles that raise the eyebrows could help too. Get an opinion from a cosmetically trained dermatologist.

HOLLOWING AT THE TEMPLES

Problem: The temple area is becoming increasingly gaunt.
Best Solution: Sculptra

All of us lose fat pads to some extent in our faces as we get older, including in the temple. Those of us who are lucky enough to start with larger fat pads often don't see this much as we age. But if you started with a thinner face or you have a low body weight, then this area can become quite gaunt looking, creating an impression of premature aging.

I really became much more aware of this area when I began working with more HIV-positive patients suffering from lipodystrophy or lipoatrophy, side effects of HIV medications that cause the loss of facial fat pads. Paradoxically, this can create a gaunt, unhealthy look even while a person is getting healthier and healthier. Approved by the FDA for the treatment of lipodystrophy, Sculptra has been a godsend for this problem. Many of my patients felt that the hollowing and gaunt look was stigmatizing. Sculptra, a synthetic product, works to thicken the skin at the injection site, correcting the hollowing and creating a much more normal, rounded facial contour.

After working with my HIV patients for some time, I noticed that many of my patients who had a low body weight also had problems maintaining fat in the temple area and cheeks. Because of the cost, I wouldn't recommend opening a whole vial just to treat this area, but if you're having Sculptra injected in other areas and you have this problem, it makes sense to treat this area simultaneously. (For more information on Sculptra, see chapter 4 and the extensive discussion there in relationship to cheeks.)

THINNING HAIR AT THE TEMPLES

This is a tough problem. Many, if not all, women have some recession and thinning of the hairline in the temple area with age. How it affects our overall outlook is really a matter of degree. A little bit, most of us can tolerate just fine, but when we notice significant thinning it can really start to change the way we feel about our appearance.

The most common culprit for this is our genes. The old wives' tale says that the mother's side of the family is responsible, but scientifically both sides count. If you see thinning on your mother or father, grandparents, aunts or uncles (particularly on both sides of the family), you're much more likely to experience thinning yourself. A smaller percentage of women suffer severe thinning, not just a little on the temples and on the top but all over the head, due to genetics.

At the very least, it's worth seeing a dermatologist and getting a medical evaluation to make sure there aren't other underlying causes or contributing factors to the problem. There are many medical causes of thinning hair, though most, but not all, cause thinning all over the scalp rather than just in certain areas.

Alopecia areata is one exception where patients often lose hair in patches. Other medical causes of hair loss include thyroid problems, low iron stores, chronic illnesses, and even protein malabsorption from diseases like celiac sprue. Acute illnesses involving a high fever or pneumonia can also cause short-term hair loss. And, of course, most women's hair gets thicker during pregnancy and then falls out in the six months after delivery.

Treatments

Options for treatment include the following.

Rogaine (over-the-counter product).   Rogaine is a relatively inexpensive, clear liquid that works fairly well in women. When put on the scalp once or twice a day, it maintains hair, and in some cases, increases hair growth. Some studies show it working better in women than in men! Though the directions say to apply it twice a day, most women I know can't stand to do that and apply it only at night, rinsing it out in the morning. Be sure to let it dry well or dry it with a hair dryer after applying. If it gets onto your pillow and then onto your face at night, you may find that you're getting increased hair growth on your face. This happens more often with the higher-strength 5 percent solution.

Hair extensions and weaves.   Many cities now have hair experts at higher-end salons who are skilled at weaving natural-looking hair into existing hair to create a thicker, natural look. For many women, these have long been an option for general styling. They do require some maintenance because the weave will grow out and need to be redone.

Hair transplants.   Just like for men, hair can be transplanted from the thicker areas around the base of the scalp into the thinner areas of the temple and the top of the head. This is a surgical procedure. The techniques have improved quite a bit over the last ten years. A natural look is generally obtainable.

Wigs and hairpieces.   Hairpieces can be matched to your own hair and are best for thinning on the top of the head. Wigs are most useful for hair loss postchemotherapy or on occasion with very severe male-pattern loss. Prices vary but not much maintenance is needed. Celebrities also seem to love these and some have a whole wardrobe of them.

THE BOTTOM LINE

- Great Botox should be virtually undetectable. You should look relaxed and natural. Frown lines and horizontal lines improve dramatically with Botox.
- Pay attention to your eyebrow position. Forehead Thermage is a relatively inexpensive, noninvasive method for treating drooping brows if the drooping is mild to moderate.
- Horizontal forehead and scrunch lines at the top of the nose respond best to Botox. Make sure your doctor or nurse is cautious with the levels—too much in your forehead, and the eyebrows may drop down.
- Very hollow temples? Sculptra works best.
- If you have hair loss, see your dermatologist for a medical evaluation.
- If you have a problem after any cosmetic treatment, call your doctor or nurse immediately and give them the opportunity to correct the problem. Many problems can easily be corrected.

4

YOUR EYES

The eyes are the windows to the soul.

Our eyes are windows—they reveal our sadness, tears, anger, joy, laughter, and desires. When first introduced to someone, we shake hands and look each other in the eye. Even beyond first impressions, our eyes convey an awful lot of information about us and who we are.

Perhaps eliminating wrinkles in your forehead was first on your list of makeover objectives, and you're now moving on to the next area: your eyes. Or, maybe you don't have a single forehead line but you're bothered by the skin around your eyes. If so, this chapter is for you. Here are some of the questions and comments I hear every week:

- "How can I improve my crow's feet?"
- "I hate this crinkly skin around my eyes."
- "Is there any way to get rid of these bags under my eyes without surgery?"
- "I feel like I look tired all the time."

Whether the problem is crow's feet, crinkly skin around the lids, or permanent bags under the eyes, many women feel their eyes look older, more stressed, or more tired than they feel. In this chapter we'll look at treatments that can help the appearance of your eyes match your spirit.

CURES FOR CROW'S FEET OF ALL DEPTHS AND SIZES

Problem: Lines that radiate out from the outer edges of the eye
Best Solutions: Quick fix—Botox or CosmoPlast/Cosmoderm; long term—fractional or traditional resurfacing laser or a long-wave collagen-building laser

Sometimes I wonder who was the nice person who thought up a crow's foot in the first place to describe these little (and sometimes big) lines that radiate out from the eyes. I like to think of these instead as smile lines. Surely, some movement around the eyes when we smile is a good thing since none of us wants that Oscar-night freeze look!

Many of my patients in their fifties or sixties tell me that they don't mind having some lines radiating out from their eyes. They don't want these lines eliminated completely, but they wish they weren't quite so

---

MAKE A LIST OF WHAT IS BOTHERING YOU! HERE'S A START:

- upper eyelids or lower eyelids or both
- crow's feet
- sagging and excess skin
- crepey texture
- hollow under-eye area
- fat pads right under the eye
- bags over the cheekbones
- dark circles under the eye

---

deep or noticeable. The truth is, we've come by some of these lines honestly, through joyous activities like smiling and expressing our emotions throughout our lives. But for many women, once the lines start to look more like small crevices, or extend way down onto the cheek area, they become bothersome.

When I assess my patients' skin, I often rank crow's feet as shallow (barely visible nonsmiling), moderate (can see definite crow's feet with the face not smiling), and deep (more like a groove that extends down onto the cheek).

Short-Term Fixes

Many women are looking for short-term fixes for their crow's feet, in other words a makeover that will get them results within one week. Here are solutions that can provide that quick help:

Eye creams.   If you aren't already, use an eye-area moisturizer morning and night and an eye-area sunscreen every morning like Dermalogica Total Eye Care SPF 15 or the Colorescience My Favorite Eyes Cream (22 percent zinc). As for eye creams before bed, there are several good ones. If you don't already have a favorite, try SkinCeuticals Eye Balm, La Mer Eye Balm, or SkinWithin Eyebright. Just using a moisturizer, if you haven't been, helps because the skin around the eye has very few oil glands.

WHAT CAUSES CROW'S FEET?

- sun damage to collagen
- muscle movement, like smiling and squinting
- loss of fullness in the upper cheeks with aging
- fewer elastic fibers—sagging

Botox.   Botox takes about five days to work after it's injected, relaxing the muscles around your eyes that cause crow's feet lines. Such treatments can be customized for you, using less or more Botox depending on whether you're going for a more natural look or no movement at all around the eyes. Usually three or four small injections are made where the wrinkles appear. Typically, there is little to no bruising afterward. To minimize bruising, just be sure to use no aspirin, ibuprofen, or Aleve for one week prior to treatment.

Fillers: CosmoDerm and CosmoPlast.   You can also get a nice result instantly by filling crow's feet with Cosmoplast or CosmoDerm (collagen). Restylane and Juvederm (hyaluronic acid) are thicker and have a greater tendency to be lumpy around the eyes, but the thinner "fine line" forms might be okay. If not injected perfectly, annoying lines or ridges can form at the site. CosmoDerm is better for fine to medium lines and CosmoPlast for deeper ones. With an experienced doctor or nurse, you can get a nice smooth fill of the lines without bumps.

Using both Botox and CosmoDerm.   If you have deep lines, you'll get the best results if you opt for both together, though that can get expensive (Botox and filler cost about a thousand dollars). The filler acts to plump up the lines while the Botox relaxes the muscles that cause the lines in the first place.

The problem with Botox and fillers around the eye area is that the procedures need to be repeated two to four times a year—usually more the first year and less after that. Many of my long-term patients come twice a year. But laser treatments can give longer-term results.

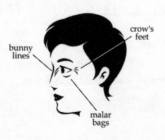

TERMS YOU'LL WANT TO KNOW

- *crow's feet*: the lines that radiate out like spokes from a wheel from the outer corner of your eye
- *bunny lines*: the lines that come down the side of your nose when you squint hard or wrinkle your nose
- *malar bags*: the puffiness that occurs over the bone directly under the eye
- *orbicularis muscle*: the muscle that runs all the way around the eye that allows you to open your eyes wide or squint, etc.

Longer-Term Fixes

Lasers can offer longer-term results because they build up your own collagen in and around the wrinkles by stimulating your cells to make more collagen. Let's consider the four main options.

Fractional lasers.   These newer lasers like the Fraxel may prove to be better than the long-wave lasers, but there isn't as much data on them yet. They use tiny, microscopic laser beams to remove older collagen and replace it with new (think aerating your lawn). They build collagen to help you reduce wrinkles. Generally, makeup can be used for cover-up, and downtime is minimal.

Resurfacing lasers.   Because we now have better options, I no longer recommend older, carbon-dioxide or erbium resurfacing lasers for work around the eyes. If only the eye area is treated, it can result in a kind of a raccoon-like look, where the eye area is permanently white and the skin oddly shiny. In other words, there can be a mismatch between your regular skin and the skin that has been resurfaced. Better is a lighter erbium laser. But, even with that, the skin around the eye can have a different texture if it's done deeply. These lasers are usually best used on the full face and not just on one area.

Collagen-building (long-wave) lasers for crow's feet.   With virtually no downtime after the procedure, these lasers (CoolTouch, Aramis, Smoothbeam) can give you a nice result over time, if you're *patient.* It may take six to nine months before you notice any significant change. Most women usually need a series of five to six treatments, followed by maintenance twice a year. But the advantage of these lasers is that you may be able to reduce or eliminate the use of injectables, which for many women is a nice plus. The laser can leave a little redness for a few days, easily covered by makeup.

Risks of Fillers

The risks of the safe fillers like Juvederm, Restylane, or CosmoPlast are the same as with any injectable—bruising, puffiness, lumpiness, and very rare allergic reactions. Feel the bone around your eye socket. This is called the orbital bone. Fillers should always be injected over or outside the orbital bone. The minute you go inside the orbital bone near the eyeball, there are a slew of other risks involving the eye itself. Don't allow any practitioner to inject around the eyes unless he or she is an expert.

Laser Safety

Most lasers are safe to use in the eye area as long as proper eye protection is used and the laser is aimed over or outside the bony orbital rim, not over the eyeball itself. Any side effects are usually short term, including puffiness, an occasional bruise, or a superficial blister. There have been some rare cases of permanent damage to the eye when proper eye protection was not used or the wrong type of laser was used too close to the eye (see the regional guide for laser centers in your area, run by board-certified dermatologists with experience and expertise in laser work). Avoid medi-spas and mall laser clinics, where the laser "technicians" often have no formal medical training, have taken only a two- or three-day training seminar, and, depending on state laws, do not get on-site supervision by a laser-trained physician.

REAL-WORLD ADVICE

What is the most cost-effective way to treat crow's feet?   If you can do only one thing, I would start with Botox. If you like the effect from the Botox, maybe eventually consider doing some of the collagen-building laser treatments after Botox.

When would a collagen-building laser be better than a resurfacing laser and vice versa?   It may turn out in a few years that the new fractional resurfacing lasers are the perfect answer to deeper crow's feet, but that remains to be proven. So if you have a center experienced with both traditional and fractional resurfacing and long-wave lasers, go there for advice.

I'm in my early thirties. Is there any way to prevent crow's feet later on?   Yes, some of the problem with crow's feet is sun damage and can be prevented by using sunscreen daily to prevent damage to your collagen and elastic fibers. Always wear an eye-area sunscreen. Also, there are very few oil glands around the eyes, so use an eye cream at night to moisturize the area. Depending on your age, you may want to also apply an antioxidant, like the SkinCeuticals Vitamin C E Ferrulic and a vitamin-A cream like Renova. And be sure to always wear sunglasses to minimize squinting. Crow's feet come from squinting and sun damage, primarily.

My doctor injected Restylane in my crow's feet and it got all lumpy.   Your doctor probably used a Restylane that's too thick for the thin skin around the eyes. I would recommend that only Restylane Fine Line (available only in Canada) or injectables like CosmoDerm or Cosmo-Plast be used in the crow's-feet area. Also, make sure your doctor or nurse is very experienced. Even when using the correct product, it can be difficult to get this area absolutely smooth.

I don't like the idea of Botox. Can I get the same result with a filler for my crow's feet?   Nothing but Botox will relax the muscles that are causing the scrunching when you smile. That said, filling in the lines may give you an appearance that is almost as nice. You could always try the filler first and if you don't like the results, try Botox as a second option. The good thing about Botox is that if you don't like it or don't want to continue using it, you can just let it wear off (about three to five months) and not go back. Or, opt for lasers, but remember it takes much longer to see a result.

UPPER EYELIDS

Problem: Sagging and crinkly upper-eyelid skin
Best Solutions: Eyelid Thermage or surgery (blepharoplasty)

One of my patients described feeling as if her eyebrows were sitting on her upper eyelids. I often hear it described as a "heavy" feeling. Another woman told me she felt as if she couldn't see—and she couldn't! The hooding (that excess flap of upper-eyelid skin) had become so bad (she was in her sixties) that the extra flap of skin was cutting off her peripheral vision on both sides.

Hooding or Saggy Upper-Eyelid Skin

This problem almost always runs in families. Surgery may be your best option, but if the hooding is just beginning and is minimal, you may be able to correct the problem with eyelid Thermage, the sound wave (radio frequency) technology that is best known for tightening the skin on the face. In 2006, Thermage came out with a quarter-centimeter tip specifically for the eyelid, which is FDA approved. This tiny little Thermage tip, designed for use on the very thin skin of the eyelids, can be used right up to the eyelid margin safely. This is not eyelid surgery—I repeat, this is not eyelid surgery—and the results are not as dramatic, but without surgery and without any downtime you can get a subtle but noticeable tightening around the eyelid area. If this treatment is combined with forehead Thermage, which lifts the eyebrows a bit, then it makes the eyes look more open and the skin tighter.

Eyelid Thermage.   When you go to your doctor for eyelid Thermage, make sure he or she takes a good medical eye history, including questions about prior eye surgeries, glaucoma, ocular rosacea, and other pertinent conditions.

Here's how the procedure unfolds. First you remove any contact lenses and makeup. Then, a small rubber patch (grounding pad) will be placed on your abdomen. A small numbing drop is put in the eye itself (just like at the eye doctor) and a special contact lens shield is placed in the eye. The contact lens shield has a cushion of special ointment on the side next to the eye. You can feel the lens, but it's not uncomfortable at all.

Then, the doctor will place the tiny tip on the eyelid skin and go over it pulse by pulse. Multiple passes are done, all over the eyelid skin right up to the eyelid margin, up to the eyebrows, and down to the eye socket bone. You may feel a sensation of heat, but again, it is not uncomfortable. If you do feel discomfort, ask your nurse or doctor to turn the energy down just a bit.

You'll notice some immediate tightening of the skin and a bit of puffiness, unnoticeable to anyone else, immediately after the procedure. But there shouldn't be bruising or redness of any kind. With Thermage, you can put on your makeup and go right back to work. (I've done this myself.) All together, the process takes about an hour or an hour and a half.

Most people see some subtle immediate result, and the effect becomes more noticeable gradually over the next four to six months. The cost for this procedure, depending on where you live, is usually somewhere from one thousand to two thousand dollars. Again, this procedure is best for those with early crinkling of the skin and mild hooding.

What if you're dead set against surgery?   Some of my patients who have moderate to severe hooding, but are absolutely against any type of plastic surgery, have asked me if eyelid Thermage could help. I counsel them that they can certainly try it, though they should understand that they may not get the results they're hoping for. Also, they may need two to four treatments. Some of my patients have now done two or three treatments about four to six months apart and have gotten nice results. I would still caution anyone with moderate to severe hooding that this might not be money well spent.

Surgical options.   This is one area where I think surgery is often the best option. Upper-eyelid surgery in the hands of a good, experienced surgeon is quite straightforward, complications are rare, and the results are often beautiful. If you have moderate to severe hooding, surgery could be the best course. The downtime is usually one to two weeks, depending on how much bruising you have. Cost, depending on region, ranges from four thousand to ten thousand dollars.

Crinkly Upper-Eyelid Skin

Those tiny, fine lines on the eyelids are one of the tougher problems to solve on the upper eyelid. The eyelid Thermage mentioned above helps some, but doesn't offer a complete fix. Also, the Fraxel laser has a small tip that can be used on the brow bone and eyelid itself, which may be helpful. If you have excess skin, of course, eyelid surgery, as outlined above, may help.

Other options include peels, the Fraxel laser, and light resurfacing lasers like the erbium laser. Please remember, only an expert, board-certified dermatologist or plastic surgeon should be working around your eye area. A moderate peel or resurfacing laser can work well if it's done right, but the potential for complications, scarring, infection, and other issues is more than with eyelid Thermage or eyelid Fraxel laser. Expert cosmetic dermatologists only, please.

REAL-WORLD ADVICE

I'm forty-three, and really don't want surgery, but I have a lot of hooding already, and it runs in my family. What would you advise? This is one area where surgery, in the hands of an excellent plastic surgeon, may be the best option. With relatively little downtime, the surgery usually has excellent results and minimal risk. If it were me, I'd probably have the surgery and then use eyelid Thermage to maintain my improvement every other year or so. Even with an excellent surgery, the results tend to last only about five to ten years. Eyelid Thermage may help you avoid a second surgery. Or, you could choose the eyelid Thermage but understand you may need to do several treatments and may not be completely happy with it.

I'm not sure what products to use on my eyelids. They seem to be really sensitive.   You're not imagining this. The eyelid skin *is* more sensitive because it's so thin. Products that you may tolerate just fine on other parts of your body may cause a reaction on your eyelids. My recommendation is to use products that are specially formulated for the eyelid. If you're very sensitive, you may want to look into products like the Free & Clear line, marketed as Vanicream. This line is free of many of the additives that seem to irritate most people. Most of my patients who are prone to allergies and eczema do well with this product line. If you can't find Vanicream, look for products with short ingredient lists, minimal preservatives, and avoid fragrances and lanolin.

Personally, I love many of the organic and "natural" lines that are being sold now. But, surprisingly, if you have a lot of allergies, these are not always good choices. The plant extracts and essential oils they contain can be very irritating for the allergy prone. For sun protection, I highly recommend the Colorescience My Favorite Eye Cream (22 percent zinc) or Dermalogica Total Eye Protection SPF 15 Eyelid Sunscreen, both mineral-titanium-based sunscreens that contain no chemicals.

If I decide I want surgery, how do I find a good surgeon?   If you have a good board-certified dermatologist, ask him or her. Chances are that he or she has referred to the plastic surgeons in the area and will know their work intimately. But if you don't, you may want to ask other doctors or friends for a starting point. I always recommend talking to at least two or three plastic surgeons before you opt for treatment and decide on your doctor. Even experts will have different approaches or may have different advice. It's important to have a surgeon whom you feel comfortable talking to and who will answer your questions generously. If the surgery goes perfectly, it isn't so much of an issue, but if you have any type of complication you will want to have someone with whom you can communicate easily and whom you trust. (See chapter 16 on how to find a good doctor.)

LOWER EYELIDS, UNDER-EYE BAGS, AND THE AREA UNDER THE EYE

The lower eyelid is a much more complicated area to treat than the upper eyelid, and surgeries go wrong here more often than on the upper eyelid. If you decide that surgery is your best option, be very careful to pick an excellent surgeon for this operation. Complications that can occur from surgery here include an eyelid that won't close properly due to the lower-eyelid skin being pulled too tightly. If this occurs, the eye itself will dry out from constant exposure to the air, particularly at night, and in turn this can cause corneal problems. Also, in the past, some surgeons took out too much fat under the eye which, over time, led to a hollow, bony look in the under-eye area. Scarring can also be an issue.

Eye creams.   There is no eye cream that will fix anything more than dry skin and help with very fine lines on the eyelids. They won't fix under-eye bags or loose skin. The ones that claim to tighten the skin may work for a few hours but that's it.

Puffiness Right Under the Eye

If you have a true fat pad underneath the eye causing the puffiness, non-surgical treatments will not work. However, if the problem is due to a little excess skin and it is not too severe, then the eyelid Thermage procedure discussed in the upper-eyelid section may be helpful for you. You'll need a dermatologist to help you figure out which it is.

The following factors can all affect puffiness under the eyes:

Allergies.   Remember that all kinds of external issues can affect the delicate eyelid skin. If you have allergies and are constantly rubbing your eyes, or if you have a dust mite problem in your pillows, mattress, and bed linens, do not have any kind of surgery until you have controlled this

WHY SHOULD I USE A SPECIAL
EYELID SUNSCREEN?

- Many of the wrinkles around your eye are caused by sun damage.
- Regular sunscreen used on the eyelids causes irritation and allergic reactions.
- You can get moisturizer and skin protection all in one.
- Dermalogica Total Eyecare SPF 15 or Colorescience My Favorite Eyes Cream (22 percent zinc) are good choices. Order at www.skintour.net.

problem. Why spend all that money only to undo it in the next year or so with recurrent allergy problems? If you're not sure if you have a dust-mite allergy, see an allergist who will test you and give you resources to protect yourself from dust mites. It really does help!

Crying.   Crying will make this area puffy as well. One of my patients, who was going through a divorce and (very understandably) crying frequently, complained about her eyelid puffiness to me. In this situation, using some ice bags or a bag of frozen peas for five or ten minutes may be helpful. In addition, sleeping with your head on an extra pillow will help in that fluid won't accumulate as much in your eye area overnight. For puffiness due to external factors, make sure to apply a very light moisturizer around the eye. Sometimes a very heavy moisturizer stretches the tissue even more.

Salt and fluid intake.   Salt and fluid intake really affect this area. Particularly as we get older, the fluid that accumulates in our lower legs during the day reequilibrates to our face at night. If you drink lots of water, minimize salt intake and sleep on an extra pillow. This will help lessen the eyelid puffiness. Some of my patients have noticed that if they drink alcohol, they feel as if their eyes are puffy in the morning. If you've had a wild night, try drinking a lot of water, and maybe even take a B vitamin before going to bed.

Looking Hollow Under the Eyes

Most of the time, a very hollow under-eye socket is a genetic tendency. Everyone has some mild loss of the fat pad under their skin as they get older. This is most noticeable in the lower under-eye area (also called the tear trough), and usually starts in our forties or early fifties. Fat pads around the eye area can also slip a bit. A fat pad that was higher up may gradually move down with the effects of gravity and time.

Weight loss.   Weight loss affects fat all over your body, including your face. Fat pads are fascinating, because different areas are metabolically active at different times of our lives. As time goes on, some fat pads tend to increase while others tend to decrease. The fat pads in our faces tend to decrease over time—darn!—as opposed to those in our abdomen. If you've lost weight recently, that might be the reason that you're looking more hollow around the eyes.

Eyelid surgery.   One of the common causes I've seen for a hollowed, bony look around the eyelids is blepharoplasty, or lower-eyelid surgery. In the past, surgeons would remove fat from around the eye area

---

WHY DO I HAVE DARK CIRCLES?

- genetics
- dehydration
- lack of sleep, illness
- too much fat around the eye removed at eyelid surgery

in younger women, leaving them at risk for an unpleasant, hollow appearance ten or fifteen years later. If that has occurred, you may want to look into fillers like Restylane and Juvederm or Sculptra, which can build the collagen, or look into fat transplantation around the eye, a procedure in which some fat from another part of your body is transplanted into the eye area. Please see the regional resource section. There are only a few centers in the country where there are experts experienced enough to do fat transplantation under the eye area well.

Solutions for Under-Eye Hollows

Patients often ask me why fat isn't used more often as a filler. It's a great question. If it worked well, it would be such a perfect solution, because there would be no risk of any type of adverse reaction. There are some experts in the country who do an excellent job of it, but they are few and far between. The problem with using fat as a filler is that the results are often unpredictable. The effect can be lumpy and the longevity is widely variable—in some people it will last many years with a nice result, and in others it will be gone in six months. You also risk a lot of bruising and puffiness with fat transplantation around the eye area, often necessitating two or three weeks of downtime. It's also expensive compared to some of the other fillers.

Restylane and Juvederm.   If done by an expert injector, this is *probably* safe. But there isn't enough safety data on Restylane in the under-eye area to be absolutely sure it's safe. The concern is that a blood vessel could be blocked with the thick gel, and blindness could occur. It may be wise to wait until it's been proven to be safe. Since Restylane is a cosmetic procedure and the loss of an eye is a disastrous complication, until there is a study proving its safety, it may be wise to wait.

Sculptra.   The same safety concerns apply to Sculptra around the eye area. Dr. Vleggar of Switzerland, the world's expert on Sculptra, has treated more than four thousand patients and performed over ten thousand treatments (usually three to four per patient), frequently including the under-eye area. However, there are few injectors as expert as Dr. Vleggar. To date, there have been no reported cases of problems with eyesight after injecting Sculptra around the eye area.

Sculptra injections work to fill in the hollowness under the eyes by stimulating the growth of your body's own collagen. But Sculptra can be very slow to take effect. When the injections are done every eight weeks, the concentration is kept low, and the massaging technique that the patient does after the injections is done religiously, then a very nice result can be achieved over time.

Visible Sculptra bumps have been reported, and they can take a long time to go away in this area. But Sculptra is not for those who lack patience or who want fast results. A caveat: Expert injectors only, please.

While Sculptra has full approval in the European union and Canada, it has limited FDA approval in the United States. It can be used around the eye area as an "off-label" use only. Full approval is pending in 2008.

Crinkly Skin Under the Eye

One of my patients nailed this when she said that what really bothers her is that her makeup gets stuck in all the cracks around her eyes. Now that I am in my 50s, I know exactly what she means. Just as with crinkly skin on the upper eyelids, the best non-surgical choices are eyelid Thermage or Fraxel laser, and possibly a light resurfacing laser or a peel.

Eyebags over the Cheekbones (Malar Bags)

This is a different problem from bags right under the eye. Bags that occur near the bone or down on to the cheek can be caused by one of three different things, or a combination of all three—*excess skin, fat-pad slippage,* or *loosening of the muscle under the eye* (orbicularis oculi muscle).

The treatment depends on which problem you have. Look in the mirror. You can determine if you have excess skin by taking your finger and lightly pulling up on the skin under the eye. Does the bag seem to correct? This isn't foolproof. You may be pulling the muscle up also, but, if it's just excess skin, you should be able to move the skin lightly over the underlying structures and see it correct. So how to fix this? If your problem is excess skin, and the problem is minimal, then the eyelid Thermage may be enough. If the excess skin is moderate to severe, then plastic surgery is your best option.

If one of the fat pads that should be inside the eye socket has slipped down over or slightly under the bone, then you should be able to feel a soft fatty deposit there. This is tricky, so if you aren't sure, you might need your doctor to help you figure it out. If the fat pads have slipped, then surgery will be best. I wouldn't recommend even trying the eyelid Thermage.

For the third possibility, that the orbicularis oculi muscle itself has loosened over time, try this: Tilt your head slightly back and squint into the mirror. If it's the muscle, you should see the muscle tighten and move up, and the whole area will look improved. It can sometimes be a combination of the above and so if you're not sure, you may need a consultation from a good cosmetic dermatologist or plastic surgeon. If the orbicularis oculi is too loose, you may need surgery.

An eye-muscle exercise.   However, you could first try this eye-muscle exercise: Pull the skin tight around your eyes first, so that the muscle action doesn't aggravate your wrinkles. Then, do that tightening exercise (described above) twenty-five or thirty times to see if you can increase the tone in that muscle. Do that every day for a month. The evidence for this working is entirely anecdotal, but I think it's worth a try for a couple of months if it might save you a surgery.

Allergies also aggravate this problem. If you're unsure, please see your allergist for testing. Controlling dust mites and other allergens in your environment will almost always help improve puffiness around the eyes if it's allergy related.

REAL-WORLD ADVICE

Can under-eye bags be prevented?   If the problem is fat pads, no. If the problem is excess skin, using a daily eyelid sunscreen (which prevents damage to the elastic and collagen fibers of the thin eyelid skin) and controlling allergies will help. If you're in your late thirties or early forties, you might want to consider using the eyelid Thermage technique once a year or every other year for preventive maintenance. There is no data on this, but because the procedure is safe, has no downtime, is virtually painless, and not too expensive, it's a logical option to consider.

I've been using Botox in my crow's feet area for many years, and I think it might be making my under-eye bags worse. Is this possible? I've never seen a study on this, but after years of experience, I do think that this happens occasionally. My professional guess is that this could occur because the orbicularis oculi muscle, which is the muscle that runs all the way around the eye, is relaxed when Botox is done. In some people, I think that the lower portion of the same muscle seems to relax a little bit too much, possibly because patients with Botox do not squint as much (squinting activates the muscle). If you think this might be happening, try stopping the Botox and doing the orbicularis oculi (eye muscle) exercise suggested above for a few months and see if it improves. If not, it's probably not the Botox.

Are there any creams that really work for under-eye bags? No, unfortunately, there are not. There are some that can make a temporary improvement in the under-eye area (for a few hours at most), but no cream that I know of permanently improves under-eye bags.

Why does my under-eye area always look puffy in the morning? The fluid in our legs equalizes at night and redistributes to our faces as we lie prone in bed. Also contributing are excess salt intake, excess cheap carbs (like white sugar, white flour, and alcohol), allergies, and crying. Try drinking lots of water during the day, limiting your salts and cheap carb intake, sleeping on an extra pillow at night, and controlling your allergies.

My doctor injected Sculptra under the eyes, and I now have lumps there. What should I do? If you've finished your Sculptra injection series and the bumps are small, massage them gently with lotion for five minutes twice a day. They should gradually dissipate on their own. If they're visible at all or seem to be getting larger, or if you've done the massage for two weeks and it's still not getting any better, then call your doctor. He or she can inject a small amount of sterile saline or an antiinflammatory solution (Kenalog) right into the Sculptra bump to break it up. You'll still need to massage once or twice a day until the bump is gone. Sometimes this needs to be repeated a couple of times to get rid of the bump.

THE BOTTOM LINE

- If you don't have a problem around your upper and lower eyelids yet, then do the preventive measures—daily eyelid sunscreen, wear sunglasses to avoid squinting, control your allergies, and pay attention to dietary habits that make you retain water such as too much salt and too much white sugar and flour (cheap carbs). Consider doing eyelid Thermage every one to two years starting in your midthirties to early forties.
- If the eyelid skin is hooding or sagging and the problem is mild or even moderate, then try the nonsurgical eyelid Thermage coupled with a forehead Thermage to lift the eyebrows as well. If the problem is more one of crepey textured skin, then consider the Fraxel laser or a gentle eyelid erbium or carbon dioxide laser resurfacing.
- If your hooding or eyelid sagging is moderate or severe, you should definitely consider surgery. Consider surgery also if you have fat pads under the eye or fat pads that have slipped down over the eye socket bone. If you do decide on surgery, pick your surgeon carefully!—particularly for lower eyelid surgery, which is much trickier than the upper eyelid. Make sure you have an absolutely stellar surgeon so you don't have complications that make you look worse.

5

YOUR LIPS AND THE AREA AROUND THEM

Everything has beauty, but not everyone sees it.
—*Confucius*

Our lips and lower faces convey so much expression! After forty-plus years of gabbing, sipping, munching, laughing, and kissing, this area is likely starting to show some significant wear and tear. Marionette lines tracing from mouth to chin, curved lines running from nose to mouth, and thinning, down-turned lips: these are often the early banes of our forty- or fifty-year-old faces.

When we look at each other, the first thing we notice after the eyes are the lips. If we can make the lips and eyes look more rested and youthful, we can change the appearance of the whole face. The lips and the area around them are often the next thing patients mention to me on their makeover wish list.

If you were a fly on the wall of my exam rooms, you would hear these concerns, among others:

- "These lines around my mouth make me look old."
- "Can I make my lips just a little fuller but still look natural?"
- "I hate these lines on my upper lip. Can you make them go away?"
- "I feel like I have parentheses around my mouth."

Many of these problems can be remedied. But before you read on about how to improve these areas, ask yourself what's really bothering you about your lips or mouth. Plastic surgery can be great for jowls or sagging skin, but it does almost nothing for upper-lip lines or thin lips. It would be unfortunate to spend fifteen to twenty-five thousand dollars on a facelift only to realize that it didn't correct the one thing that bothers you the most.

SOFTENING THE LINES FROM YOUR NOSE TO YOUR MOUTH (NASOLABIAL FOLD)

Problem: The lines from my nose to my mouth are too deep
Best Solutions: Restylane and Juvederm or Sculptra

You'll sometimes see these lines referred to as parentheses or, medically, the nasolabial fold (NLF). This is one of the easiest problems to correct for most women. Unless the lines are very deep, we can fill and

---

MAKE A LIST OF WHAT IS BOTHERING YOU!
HERE'S A START:

- upper-lip lines
- lines from nose to mouth
- lines from mouth to chin
- lips shrinking
- upper and lower lips not in proportion
- fading lip outline
- lips turning down
- bumpy chin

soften these lines with a few injections of a filler like Restylane or Juvederm (hyaluronic acids).

Restylane and Juvederm

Hyaluronic acid (HA) is a natural sugar that occurs in the skin and is made synthetically in a laboratory in Sweden (Restylane) or France (Juvederm). Restylane and Juvederm contain no human or animal DNA. They are the best injectable forms because they have the best safety profiles—and they work. Millions of women worldwide have had safe HA injections. On average, the results last four to nine months, with maintenance about two visits a year. Costs can run from five hundred to fifteen hundred dollars to treat the NLF, depending on how many syringes you need to get a good correction and where you live—New York City is more expensive than Seattle, for example. The downside for HA injections is that you might experience some discomfort on injection as well as possible bruising or temporary lumpiness.

Sculptra

These lines can also be lifted and filled with injections of Sculptra. Sculptra is a newer and longer-lasting filler than Restylane and Juvederm. It has a good safety profile (but not as good as Juvederm or Restylane) if injected correctly.

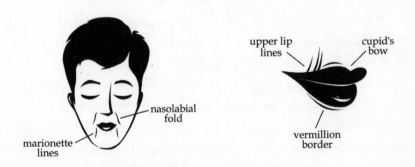

TERMS YOU'LL WANT TO KNOW

- *nasolabial fold:* the lines that look like parentheses from the nose to the mouth
- *melolabial lines:* also called marionette's lines, lines from the mouth to the chin
- *vermillion border:* the rim of the lips where it meets the skin
- *cupid's bow:* the curvy line at the center of the upper lip
- *upper-lip lines:* those pesky vertical lines or wrinkles that lipstick bleeds into

Sculptra is a type of synthetic lactic acid (poly-L-lactic acid) that stimulates collagen growth deep in the skin. You might want to start with a more temporary product like Restylane or Juvederm to make sure you like the effect on your NLF. Sculptra is longer lasting (about one to two years) and requires a series of two to four treatments four to eight weeks apart followed by approximately one maintenance treatment a year. Costs range from about six hundred to two thousand dollars per treatment. Most patients find it more comfortable than Restylane to have injected because it stings less and has a numbing agent (lidocaine) mixed in with it.

While Sculptra has full approval in Europe and Canada, it has limited FDA approval in the United States (HIV only—other uses are "off-label"). Full approval is pending in 2008.

Is Sculptra safe? Since 2003, Dr. Daniel Vleggar in Switzerland and Dr. Ute Bauer in Italy, the world's experts on Sculptra, have done more than fifteen thousand injections combined. Only about ten patients experienced problems that were visible. Even these complications were temporary—lasting less than two years. However, you want an expert cosmetic dermatologist to inject Sculptra, since it's much trickier to inject correctly than Restylane and Juvederm.

Different Filler Choices

If you look in any magazine, you'll see a new filler every month and you may wonder if it's better than those mentioned here. The simple answer is it's not. And here's why: The test of time. Many of the new fillers on the market work pretty well and may even cost less. But I strongly vote for fillers that have the best safety profiles and have been proven over time. Why take a risk on your face when there are proven, tried and true products? Even if some doctor is offering a "special" for fifty to a hundred dollars less, it hardly seems worth the risk.

Temporary or Permanent Fillers—The Pros and Cons

When you begin using a filler, always start with a temporary filler like an HA (Restylane and Juvederm). That way if you don't like the results, you won't be stuck with them forever. Make sure that you like the effect that you get and that you trust your doctor's skill before you try any longer-lasting fillers like Sculptra or Radiesse. I never recommend the "permanent" fillers like Artefill or silicone. What if the doctor injecting makes a mistake? Allergic reactions to permanent fillers can also occur one to fifteen years after they are injected, and the reactions may be permanent—red, hard lumps in your face are not fun to live with. What's more, a permanent filler that may look great at age fifty could look terrible at age fifty-eight. Faces and weight don't stay exactly the same, and you can't easily adjust a permanent filler later. To my mind, the ideal filler would last about a year and could be adjusted annually.

Here are some other tips on using a filler like Restylane or Juvederm for nasolabial lines:

- Even children have a curve here, so don't overfill this area. If it gets too flat or, heaven forbid, convex instead of slightly concave, it doesn't look natural. If you're getting Botox treatments also, schedule some of these appointments at the same time so you don't have to make so many trips.

- Good cosmetic filler work should be undetectable after the first two to seven days, when you might have a little bruising or puffiness. You should look rested, rejuvenated, and completely natural—not overfilled, stuffed, and wooden. This includes when your face is moving and at rest. If you don't, call your doctor and ask him or her to take a look. Or, find a new doctor.
- Take it easy the first few visits. You can always call a few weeks later and say you'd like a little more. It's harder to take it out—if not impossible for some fillers. Too much Restylane/Juvederm can be dissolved with a few drops of an enzyme called hyaluronidase.

Off-Label Cosmetic Treatments

The *off-label* term signifies a medication that is FDA approved in this country but not for that particular use. If a product is being used off-label, then your doctor should notify you and that fact should be included in any consent form. You shouldn't necessarily be put off by off-label products, though. Many drugs in the United States are used off-label as research develops. Botox, for instance, was used off-label for at least ten to twelve years for cosmetic purposes in the United States before its manufacturer got FDA approval for cosmetic purposes. It had been approved for medical uses many years ago.

REAL-WORLD ADVICE

My parentheses lines are asymmetrical. Can I still use a filler like Restylane?   Yes. It's fairly easy to compensate for asymmetry and make your face more symmetrical with Juvederm or Restylane.

I have very deep grooves around my mouth. Will a hyaluronic acid filler still work?   Yes. Perlane (the thicker form of Restylane) or the thicker Juvederm Ultra Plus is best if you have deep grooves.

I had Restylane once before, and it didn't last. Why not?   It could be several things. Sometimes it takes two to three treatments to build up a base. Sometimes the doctor doesn't use enough to get a good correction, or not enough in exactly the right place.

INTELLIGENTLY FULLER LIPS

Problem: My lips are too small or are losing their fullness
Best Solutions: Restylane/Juvederm, CosmoPlast

Here's the good news. With currently available techniques, almost anyone's lips can be made fuller, more shapely, and with a rejuvenated texture. And for most people, subtly (and *subtle* is the key word) augmented lips can also look very natural, rather than blown up like overstuffed sausages. This doesn't mean that there is some magic filler that works for everyone and lasts forever. But if you have a good cosmetic dermatologist, know your goals, and understand the risks and limitations of the best fillers, you can do pretty well in filling out your lips.

How would you like your lips to look?   Here's what to ask yourself: Do I like the shape of my lips overall? Are they shaped well? If not, is it more the upper lip, or the lower lip, or both? The best upper- to lower-lip proportion in most women is with the lower lip just slightly fuller than the upper lip. The upper lip should curve slightly up at the top edge where the lip meets the skin—the vermillion border.

Look at the fullness of your lips and their proportion to your face. Are they full enough? Maybe the lower lip is fine, but the upper lip is too thin, or vice versa. Are your lips in proportion to your face as a whole? I generally vote against creating large lips in a petite face, but if you have a face with a strong nose or large eyes, then larger lips might be great.

If you're thinking about enlarging or changing your lips, try to see your face and lips like an artist. The clearer you are about what you like and don't like, the more effective your cosmetic dermatologist can be in meeting your goals.

My lips are shrinking!   Three reasons. First, your lips lose fat over time just as the rest of your face does. That loss of fat is why elderly people sometimes look gaunt and bony. The second reason is more complicated. Essentially, your lips over time lose the support of the surrounding skin as the skin loses its elasticity. The upper-lip area gets longer. We also lose bone in our jaws as we age. And third, the usual suspect—sun damage, of course!

Treatments

So, what can we do to improve your lips? Restylane and Juvederm are the best, most versatile fillers to add fullness to your lips and make subtle adjustments to their shape. Think of them as adding volume to your lips. CosmoPlast and CosmoDerm are best for defining the lip border (as opposed to adding volume) and for fine lines on the upper lip. (Collagen is a second-generation protein that contains no human or animal DNA and doesn't require allergy testing first.) Using Juvederm to define the shape can make some lips look too full at the borders and can make you look "ducky." CosmoPlast and CosmoDerm are approximately four hundred to seven hundred dollars per syringe. One syringe is usually adequate to define the borders of the lips.

The original collagens (Zyderm and Zyplast—you might even remember them) derived from a bovine source (cow) that could cause allergic reactions. They're almost never used anymore because the HAs and CosmoPlast and CosmoDerm are longer lasting and don't cause allergic reactions.

The HAs in the lips react a little differently than they do in other areas of the face. Here are the potential problems:

Puffiness.   The lips are more prone to puffiness and lumps than other areas of the face. Juvederm causes less puffiness in the lips than Restylane. If you're a "puffer," with Restylane the puffiness can be quite dramatic and require hiding out for a few days. It will subside but can be very annoying. The first time you try Restylane in the lips, have the doctor be very conservative until you see if you puff a little or a lot. Other sites are not usually a problem, just the lips.

Lumps.   HAs, such as Restylane and Juvederm, can occasionally cause temporary lumps that will smooth out over two to five days. If they're still present a week later, it's easy to fix them by either draining or injecting a drop of an enzyme (hyaluronidase) which helps to dissolve the lump. Don't suffer in silence: give your doctor a call!

Less longevity.   The lips move so much with talking, eating, kissing that the HA fillers wear out sooner here—usually two to five months instead of the typical four to nine months for other areas of the face. Restylane has a new product in Sweden (Restylane Lipps) that is reputed to last much longer and still be safe and smooth. I'm hoping we'll get it here soon.

GETTING GOOD RESULTS FROM YOUR FILLERS

Here are some tips for your fillers and communicating with your doctor well:

- If it's your first time, give yourself seven to ten days before any important social/work events. You may have bruising and a small percentage of people get *very* puffy with Restylane, especially in the lips.
- Remember, to reduce bruising, no aspirin, Advil (ibuprofen), or Aleve (naprosyn) for one week prior to injections.
- Some kind of numbing, especially if you are injecting your lips, is key to a comfortable procedure. Many offices use dental blocks. Topical numbing creams should stay on for thirty to forty minutes to be effective, so come early for pre-numbing or put the cream on at home before you come. Ask your dermatologist for advice.

Most of these problems are minor and temporary. Restylane and Juvederm are very popular for the simple reason that they safely and effectively enlarge lips and fill out wrinkles.

REAL-WORLD ADVICE

My lips are medium sized, well shaped—I'd just like to try a little fuller. Then start with one-half syringe of Restylane. If you like it, you can always go a little bigger the next time. Juvederm doesn't make a half syringe yet.

I like the size and shape of my lips, but my lip edges aren't sharp, and my lipstick is starting to bleed.   One syringe of CosmoPlast or CosmoDerm will help you define the border better and fill the small lines. Or you could consider a light-medium TCA peel of your lips with an experienced cosmetic dermatologist to improve the texture and definition. This problem is mostly due to sun damage so use sunscreen on your lips every day.

I have naturally full lips, but over time they have gotten thinner. Start with one syringe of Restylane or Juvederm. You can always get more adventurous later.

Is there anything I can do to prevent my lips from getting thinner? Again, the answer is a surprising yes! It's the small stuff that counts here. Sunscreen your lips every day! Why? Because lips have even less natural protection from villain UV radiation. The more sunlight they get, the more wrinkled they will look. I also like the Bobbi Brown small lipstick tubes with SPF 15. Also, sunlight destroys elastic fibers of the skin around the lips, causing the whole area to collapse. And take calcium and vitamin D according to nutrition guidelines to maintain the bone in your jaws. If you're fifty or older, be sure to get a baseline bone density now, especially if you have a family history of osteoporosis.

UPPER-LIP LINES

Problem: Those pesky, lipstick-ruining vertical lines

Best solutions: Short term: Botox, CosmoPlast, Restylane Fine Line (Canada). Long term: lasers (erbium, fractional resurfacing, long-wave lasers)

I and millions of other women would love it if there were a magic wand that could make these lips lines miraculously disappear without any recovery time or discomfort—guaranteed. Alas, I haven't found the magic wand yet, but several treatments can offer significant improvement. You may not get a home run on these upper- and lower-lip lines, but you can get a single, double, or triple here.

Causes

Sun damage, and, to make a long story short, motion causes these lip lines. Kissing, eating, pursing when we concentrate, drinking through a straw, talking, and, of course, smoking. Our lips are extremely active! Remember, fillers will not last as long here because there is so much movement.

Treatments

Is it okay to use Botox here?   A tiny amount of Botox in the right spots here does wonders. It helps keep existing lines from getting deeper, helps to prevent new lines, and makes any filler used here last longer. Please do not let an inexperienced doctor or nurse do this! This is one area that can go terribly wrong if done badly. It will wear off, but who wants to go around looking like they've had a stroke for three or four months?

Do lasers work for upper-lip lines?   There are three kinds of lasers for upper-lip lines: (1)collagen-building lasers (Cooltouch, Smoothbeam), which do not break the skin and therefore have little or no downtime; (2)resurfacing lasers (erbium and carbon dioxide) that take a layer of skin off and require one to two weeks to heal; and (3) Fraxel laser, a fractional resurfacing laser that heals quickly. I rarely recommend the traditional resurfacing lasers anymore because my patients can't afford the time it takes to heal properly, but they work well. The area can also remain red or pink for months, and later it may even turn a whitish color and not match the surrounding skin. If you're busy or hate using makeup, go for less downtime with the Fraxel or collagen-building lasers, even if they don't work quite as well.

Collagen remodeling and rebuilding lasers.   These are, very simply, lasers that build collagen without breaking the skin. These longer laser wavelengths penetrate more deeply into the dermis (the deeper layer where the collagen is) and stimulate cells there to make more collagen. In general, anything that builds collagen is good for your skin. What matters to you specifically is that these lasers can help reduce your upper lip lines. These treatments are usually done in a series of four to six with two to four weeks between treatments. You'll need maintenance treatments two times a year after the original series. Unless you're very lucky, these lasers won't completely eliminate the lines. This is a "double," not a home run.

LASERS FOR UPPER-LIP LINES

No downtime—collagen-building or remodeling lasers in a series of four to six treatments

- Fraxel
- CoolTouch
- Aramis
- ELOS
- Smoothbeam

With downtime (one to two weeks plus, to heal)—resurfacing lasers in a one-time treatment

- erbium
- carbon dioxide
- plasma

Costs vary widely for these, but you should expect one thousand to three thousand dollars for a series of four to six treatments around the mouth only.

Resurfacing lasers.   The Fraxel laser is a mimimal-downtime fractional-resurfacing laser. You can go back to your normal activities the next day. It also takes two to four treatments. The results are better than the long-wave lasers but not quite as good as the resurfacing lasers, which, on the other hand, can produce quite good results with one treatment. The catch, as I said above, is that the traditional resurfacing lasers (carbon dioxide and erbium) take a layer of skin off and require a good week or two to heal. Even after that, your skin can remain pink or red for several months. If you treat your upper lip or the area around the mouth only, beware of color mismatches if you tan at all or have a darker skin color.

How do I know which option to use?   First, are your wrinkles here mild (can barely see them in a candlelit restaurant), moderate (always visible but not too bad), or deep (let's face it—these are tire tracks)? Depending on your answer, consider the following:

- Mild lines. I'd recommend a few drops of Botox two to three times a year and a series of treatments with a Fraxel laser or collagen-building laser, followed by occasional maintenance treatments. Or, for an event or quick fix, CosmoPlast or CosmoDerm.
- Moderate lines. I'd recommend the fillers CosmoPlast or Cosmo-Derm, or Restylane Fine Line (Canada), a few drops of Botox two to three times a year, and then a Fraxel laser or a collagen-building laser for long-term improvement, leading to less maintenance over time.
- Deep lines. If you have the time and a good cosmetic dermatologist experienced in these lasers, go for the erbium or carbon-dioxide laser. If you don't have the former, then just know you'll need quite a bit of maintenance with the options above.

Warning: Don't let anyone inject anything permanent in small lip lines like silicone or Artefill. It can get lumpy. Sculptra is also not a good choice in the lips or lip lines. The lighter-weight HAs, like Restylane Fine Line (Canada), can be okay. But regular weight Restylane can be too puffy in these upper-lip lines. CosmoDerm or CosmoPlast in the upper lip lines are a good choice in a filler.

REAL-WORLD ADVICE

I'm just beginning to get some lines at the edge of my lips. What would you recommend?   I would use one syringe of CosmoPlast here to just outline the vermillion border. CosmoPlast can look very natural and soft, and the slight stretching will virtually erase those early lines.

I hate these lines, but I also live somewhere where it's hard to get these services, and the maintenance is too costly.   Then definitely bite the bullet, if you decide to do anything at all, and find a good dermatologic laser surgeon in the nearest large city (see the Resources section). Opt for the one-time erbium or carbon-dioxide laser. Remember—this takes two weeks to heal and can stay pink or red for months sometimes.

Which fillers work best here for upper-lip lines?   CosmoPlast is best here, or CosmoDerm, its lighter cousin. When injected with a 32- or 30-gauge needle (like acupuncture needles), it is smooth, fills well, and doesn't swell as much as the HA products (yes—even the ones for fine lines). CosmoPlast lasts longer than CosmoDerm. Costs for both CosmoPlast and the HAs are four hundred to seven hundred dollars per syringe.

MARIONETTE'S LINES

Problem: The lines from the corner of the mouth to the chin
Best solutions: Restylane and Juvederm, Sculptra, Thermage

Think of the Nutcracker and how the jaw hinges with a groove there. That's how these lines that run from the corners of your mouth down to your chin got their name.

Causes

Many women in their forties and fifties want to know why these lines are suddenly appearing or deepening on their faces. In general, there are three reasons:

First, over time you're losing the fat pads in your cheeks and lower face. The sagging pulls the skin down and toward the mouth. This is why "revolumizing" the cheeks improves these lines by lifting them up. Sculptra, which adds volume to the cheek area, can work well here. Second, the sun damage to the cheeks and around the mouth is causing the skin to lose elasticity (read sagging) here. This is why some tightening here with Thermage helps (more on this below). And third, if you have osteoporosis, bone loss in the jaw and chin is causing the same kind of problem..

Treatment

We've talked about the HAs (Restylane and Juvederm). These work well here, and usually one to three syringes will fill the area nicely, depending on your age and the number and depth of lines. Expect some mild bruising if more than one syringe is used. Costs range from four hundred to eight hundred dollars per syringe, and treatments last four to nine months depending on which HA was used and how much.

If you really need some gentle tightening throughout your whole face, including here, then I recommend a Thermage (see chapter 6) first, followed by the filler. Thermage is the sound wave (radiofrequency) that gently tightens (this is *not* a facelift) the whole cheek area, softening marionette's lines too. It works well when done correctly on the right patient, for instance, someone aged forty to sixty with mild to moderate sagging. You can go immediately back to work—and I mean immediately. I've done it! Costs for full face generally range from twenty-two hundred to three thousand dollars. It's usually repeated every one to two years depending on age.

Why should I do full-face Thermage instead of just around my mouth? Tightening over the whole face is progressive. As you tighten higher up on the face, like the forehead and upper cheeks, it in turn helps tighten the midcheek, which tightens the lower face, which tightens around the lips. The whole face gets better lift, which results in firmer looking skin and better supported cheeks, jaw line, and lips.

If you dislike the maintenance with the HAs, or you have a lot of hollowing in your cheeks, Sculptra, as mentioned above, may be a better option for you than HAs because it lasts longer. Filling hollow areas in the cheeks with Sculptra softens the Marionette's lines. Do the Thermage before the Sculptra if you're planning to do both.

RAISING THE CORNERS OF YOUR MOUTH

Problem: The corners of my lips are turning down
Best Solution: Restylane or Juvederm

Women with this problem can look sad or even angry when they feel just fine. This is easier to correct than you might think. A small amount of a filler like Restylane or Juvederm is injected at the corner of the mouth and in the fold (melolabial groove) that extends down from the corner of the mouth. This will plump that area out nicely and raise the corner. Many lips look good with the corners of the lips raised back up to level. Some lips look even more attractive with a very slight upturn at the corners (think Catherine Zeta-Jones).

Another approach is to put a small drop of Botox on a certain spot on the chin to weaken the muscle that is pulling the corner down. This is an advanced Botox technique, so don't let someone who's new to Botox try this on you.

MAKING YOUR LIPS SMOOTHER

Problem: My lips are wrinkly

Best Solutions: Antioxidant creams, fillers, light TCA peels

As we pass thirty, our lips begin to lose their smoothness and glossiness, thanks to sun damage and dryness. The goal here is to reverse both as much as possible.

If the texture of your lips seems dry and wrinkly, there are several options:

- Avoid sun damage. Use sunscreen on your lips daily and use lipsticks or lip balm with sunscreen. For lipstick with sunscreen, try the Bobbi Brown SPF 15 or Laura Mercier SPF 15.
- Hydrate. Use moisturizer on your lips morning and night.
- Extra emollients. Still dry? Try a rich oil like shea butter before bed. L'Occitane makes a good one.
- Antioxidants. SkinCeuticals Antioxidant Lip Repair will help. If your lips are still dry and scaly, you may be allergic to something. See your dermatologist.

A "lip plumper" product is different from these and can give a *temporarily* fuller and smoother appearance. These lip glosses often contain niacinamide (a vitamin) which will dilate the blood vessels in the lips a little. Others contain a mild irritant (think of rubbing a hot pepper on your lips).

Restylane and Juvederm in the lips will make the surface smoother at the same time that they plump, but they're expensive if you use them just for glossiness and texture.

If your lips are quite sun damaged, a peel can certainly help, especially if the border of your lips is getting fuzzy. You can tell this if you find it hard to see the exact outline of the lips where you would put your lipstick pencil. The lighter peels like glycolic or salicylic acid may help if done in a series. But the trichloroacetic acid or TCA peel is the best for this area. Be sure your dermatologist is experienced with this. The peel solution should be applied to the lips themselves and up over the margins. There is some downtime with this type of peel.

THE BOTTOM LINE

- Go slowly with fillers the first few visits. It's easy to add more and harder to take it out.
- For lines from your nose to your mouth—try Juvederm or Restylane. If you're over fifty, consider Sculptra.
- For your lips—for definition, use CosmoPlast, and for volume, try Juvederm.
- For those upper-lip lines, try Cosmoplast and lasers.
- For marionette's lines from the mouth to the chin, try Juvederm or Restylane, Sculptra, and sometimes Thermage.

YOUR CHEEKS

*When you have only two pennies left, buy a loaf of bread with one
and a lily with the other.*
—*Chinese proverb*

Let's be honest. What woman over the age of forty hasn't occasionally pulled up on the skin in front of her ears to tighten it—and voilà, a facelift! Many of us see aging in our cheeks as they naturally get wrinkles and move inward and down.

In my office, I hear the following kinds of comments:

- "What can I do about my wrinkles?"
- "When I lose weight, I really see it in my face now. It looks hollow."
- "My cheeks are getting saggy."

Whether what you see in the mirror has to do with sagging skin or hollowing where the cheeks begin to appear more gaunt, the good news is that there are nonsurgical options to address these problems, as well as wrinkles and more.

In fact, with a combination of Thermage to tighten the skin, Juvederm Ultra Plus, Perlane or Sculptra to restore lost volume, and lasers to help with wrinkles, a good cosmetic dermatologist can give you an *almost* facelift-like effect if there isn't too much loose skin on your jawline and neck.

**MAKE A LIST OF WHAT IS BOTHERING YOU!
HERE'S A START:**

- cheekbones not defined enough
- sagging upper cheek under the eye socket
- wrinkles on cheeks
- hollowing of the inner cheek near the lines from nose to mouth
- hollowing of the outer cheek (near the ears)

CORRECTING SAGGING CHEEKS

Problem: Cheek area is sagging, creating excess skin along the jawline

Best Solution: Juvederm Ultra Plus, Perlane or Sculptra and/or Thermage

Our cheeks change dramatically throughout our lives, from the iconic fat cheeks of babies to the thin, hollowed-out cheeks of older people in their eighties or nineties. In those intervening decades, cheeks change a lot. The baby's plump, round cheeks gradually give way to a softer, rounded contour in childhood, and in adolescence, the cheekbone area starts to differentiate more, coinciding with rapid growth. As we enter our forties and fifties, we lose the subsurface fat that gives our cheeks that smooth look. And if we haven't gained weight, our cheeks gradually thin and hollow out. The skin also begins to droop along the jawline and contributes to the lines from the nose to the mouth and around the mouth.

Causes

Here are the main causes of sagging cheeks. Most people have more than one.

Sun damage.   Much of the sagging and wrinkling on the cheeks is caused by sun damage, translating into the loss of collagen and elastic fibers in the skin through the entire cheek area. Think of collagen in your skin as the framing in your house. It provides the structural support for your skin. Think of elastic fibers as the bounce-back. As the sun damages the collagen and elastic fibers, the skin sags, wrinkles, and doesn't bounce back. It's never too late to start using a sunscreen every morning, though, as the skin will begin to repair itself if you protect it and use re-pair products.

Weight changes.   Our cheeks also fluctuate with weight differences. We all know that if we gain twenty or thirty pounds, the fat pads in our cheeks really fill out. Conversely, as we lose weight, those cheeks hollow again. This is more noticeable on many low-body-weight women, who become gaunt and hollow-looking through the cheek area as they age. As part of the normal process of aging, the fat pads in our cheeks tend to shrink compared to fat pads in other parts of our bodies. Hence the say-ing that as we get older, we have to choose between our faces and our tushes.

Genes.   Genes play a role in the basic shape of our faces and the ap-pearance of the cheeks and supporting structures. In some, the cheek-bones are broad and flat, while in others they're higher and more prominent. For example, many of my patients of Germanic background have fuller, heavier cheeks. The shape of our skulls is largely inherited, and that bony structure affects the way our fat pads and our skin change over the years as well.

What Can Help?

Thermage.   This works for mild to moderate sagging. As discussed, the Thermage procedure uses radiofrequency, a sound wave, to create a uniform heating effect in the deep layers (dermis) of the skin. This gentle heating process tightens existing collagen and stimulates the production of new collagen. The slight, immediate collagen contraction followed by subtle, gradual collagen tightening reduces wrinkles and achieves brow lifting, cheek tightening, and jawline tightening.

There are two versions of Thermage: the original version and the more current "multipass" version. In a 2007 study, fifty-seven hundred patients were surveyed at multiple clinics. With the multipass version, 87 percent observed some immediate tightening, 92 percent had tightening six months after treatment and 94 percent found that treatment results met their expectations. All patients showed an increase in collagen in biopsy studies, so even if you don't see a noticeable result, the procedure should help prevent more sagging. If you're over fifty, plan on two treatments six months apart for optimal results, then maintenance every one to two years.

There has been a lot of information and misinformation in the media about Thermage. I tell my patients who are good candidates for Thermage to think about baseball as a metaphor for the procedure. If they choose Thermage, they'll get a hit, but we don't know ahead of time whether it will be a single, double, or triple. Home runs are rare, which is why some of the before-and-after photos of Thermage treatments can be misleading.

Sculptra.   Discussed in the next section, Sculptra works to correct sagging because it fills out the lost volume in the cheeks that is partly creating the sagging (think of a deflating balloon). It also builds collagen, which helps with wrinkles.

Juvederm Ultra Plus and Perlane.   These are the thicker, longer-lasting forms of Juvederm and Restylane. They can be used to add volume instead of Sculptra but require more maintenance in the long run because they don't build collagen. They would be most helpful if you are under forty-five or need a "quick fix" if you have an upcoming event because Sculptra takes months to see the effects.

REAL-WORLD ADVICE

My cheeks have always been round and full, but now they are falling. I also have deep creases from my nose to my mouth. Would Thermage do the trick, or do I need surgery?   If you don't have much sagging at the jawline, then Thermage could work well for you. Fuller cheeks sometimes necessitate two or three Thermage treatments for maximum effect. But plan on needing a filler like Juvederm Ultra Plus in addition. The combination of Thermage to lift and tighten the cheeks and jawline with the Juvederm Ultra Plus to fill in the creases is optimal.

I have a little sagging through my cheeks. Would Thermage be helpful?   Yes, if the cause was mostly sun damage. If the problem is really more a loss of volume, Juvederm Ultra Plus, Perlane, or Sculptra might be a better choice for you. Using the combination of tightening with Thermage and adding volume back with a filler would be even better. Do the Thermage first followed by the Juvederm Ultra Plus or Sculptra.

I'm sixty-five years old. Am I too old for Thermage?   Not necessarily. If your skin is in good shape and you don't have large jowls, then Thermage may be helpful. Patients over sixty generally need two or three treatments four to six months apart, rather than just one, to optimize their results.

FILLING OUT CHEEKS THAT ARE TOO HOLLOW

Problem: hollow cheek area
Best Solution: Sculptra or fat

Every woman loses some of the rounded contour of her cheeks as she ages. Some women hollow all through the cheek area, while some lose fat and skin in front of the ears, through the midface, or even around the cheekbones.

If you lose fullness in the cheek, where will that extra skin go? It will follow the laws of gravity and collect at the jawline. Jowls are caused, in part, by a loss of volume in the cheeks.

Treatments

The two best treatment options for volume loss in the cheeks are fat transfer, the thicker, "volumizing" hyaluronic acid fillers, or Sculptra. Fat transfer involves taking fat from one part of your body, such as your thighs, and injecting it in another part, like the cheeks. Seems logical, doesn't it? It has the advantage of being completely natural, and most of us have enough fat somewhere in our bodies to donate to another site!

But here's why I don't recommend this expensive procedure. It can cause a great deal of bruising: patients often need two weeks or more off work to recover. It can also be lumpy and irregular, and the irregularities are hard to fix. It's unpredictable in terms of how long it lasts; for some patients it lasts six months and for some, many years. And there are very few doctors in the United States who do this procedure enough to be truly expert at it.

That's why I usually recommend the thicker Perlane, Juvederm Ultra Plus, or Sculptra. When injected correctly, they give a smooth, long-lasting correction requiring maintenance only every nine to twenty-four months after the initial series. They last a predictable amount of time in almost everyone. They cause very little bruising when injected (if done correctly); my patients go right back to their normal activities. Small lumps and bumps can occur but are generally easy to fix. Remember, with the hyaluronic acid filler the correction is immediate; with Sculptra the correction is slow (over six months) and is very natural looking.

However, in inexperienced hands, Sculptra can be bumpy, and the bumps can be difficult to correct. Even if it's injected correctly, the rare person can develop Sculptra bumps that are difficult to correct.

Is Sculptra safe?   Sculptra has been used in Europe since 1999. It comes in vials as a dry powder to which water and a numbing agent are added to reconstitute it. Prior to 2002, there were a number of problems reported in Europe. It was reformulated in 2002, and a different method of dilution used. Since then, its safety profile has been excellent. While Sculptra has full approval in Europe and Canada, full FDA approval in the United States is pending in 2008. Uses other than in HIV patients are "off-label."

How is Sculptra different from Restylane/Juvederm?   Sculptra adds volume to the face and thus lifts out grooves and hollows. This helps the appearance of wrinkles, because many wrinkles are created by loss of vol-

GETTING GOOD RESULTS FROM YOUR SCULPTRA

- Be patient. It takes six to nine months to see the full effect of a series of Sculptra treatments.
- Tell your doctor where you'd like more fullness.
- Avoid aspirin, ibuprofen (Motrin, Advil), and naprosyn (Aleve) for one week prior to your Sculptra treatments to avoid bruising.
- Massage according to the instructions your doctor gives you to avoid Sculptra bumps.

ume (again, think of a deflating balloon). Restylane and Juvederm, the hyaluronic-acid fillers, are injected directly into and under the wrinkles and grooves themselves to lift them out. But to fill a whole cheek with Restylane or Juvederm could take so many syringes it might be prohibitively expensive and take too much maintenance. With the thicker, longer-lasting forms of Restylane and Juvederm (Juvederm Ultra Plus and Perlane) now available, it makes sense in younger patients to use them. But Sculptra is still superior at building collagen and for older patients. Sculptra and Juvederm/Restylane can be used in combination by an expert dermatologist.

How often do I need to come for Sculptra treatments?   The treatments are done at four- to twelve-week intervals. Most people need between one and four treatments using a half vial to two vials at each treatment. I usually recommend one maintenance treatment per year after that. Results generally last two years but will be half gone at one year. It takes thirty to sixty days to see the full effect of a treatment. It lasts longer in some individuals.

Are the injections painful?   There should be little discomfort with the injections because Sculptra is mixed with lidocaine, which is a local anesthetic.

What will I look like right after a treatment?   You can put on makeup immediately (some doctors may prefer you wait a day or two) and go back to normal activities. It's best not to exercise vigorously for one to two days. There is almost undetectable fullness (from the water in the product) for about two days after a treatment. A little bruising is normal, but it's usually minimal.

Is there anyone who should not use Sculptra?   Do not use Sculptra if you are *allergic to lidocaine* or are pregnant or nursing. Do not use if you have lupus, Sjögren's syndrome, rheumatoid arthritis, or other related autoimmune diseases.

Sculptra and HIV.   Sculptra is also used for AIDS patients to correct the hollowing that comes with the medications used to treat AIDS—called retroviral agents. If you have AIDS, this problem is called lipodystrophy and can be stigmatizing. Sculptra has been used frequently to correct this problem with great results. Sculptra has been approved by the FDA for use in HIV-positive individuals only. The approval for non-HIV individuals is pending. Sculptra can be used legally as long as you sign an off-label consent form. Ethical medical practices will have you sign an off-label consent form if you are not HIV positive, until full FDA approval is received.

REAL-WORLD ADVICE

On one side of my face I look more hollow than on the other side. Is Sculptra still a good choice?   Yes. With Sculptra it is easy to correct facial asymmetries.

I had a Sculptra treatment at another office and have had problems with lumps. What should I do now?   There are several different ways to treat these bumps. First, I would call the office where you had the injections done. They should be able to instruct you in a course of self-massage of the bumps, and they might inject sterile saline into the lumps to break them up. If they seem at a loss for what to do, you might want to contact the Sculptra company through their website, and ask for the most experienced injector in your area to help you.

DEFINING AND RESTORING CHEEKBONES

Problem: Flat, sagging, or bony cheekbones
Best Solution: Juvederm Ultra Plus, Perlane, or Sculptra
   There are usually three reasons for redefining cheekbones:

   - The area is flattening with age.
   - The cheekbones are bony or gaunt looking.
   - The skin over the cheekbone is sagging.

Treatments

Juvederm and Restylane.   Juvederm and Restylane come in different molecular weights, and the thicker ones last longer. The thicker ones are called Juvederm Ultra Plus and Perlane. If you want a more subtle ef-

---

JUVEDERM AND RESTYLANE
PROS

- instant effects
- if not much correction is needed, more cost effective than Sculptra
- usually one syringe to each cheek, two syringes total
- can go fuller by using the thicker forms Perlane or Juvederm Ultra Plus
- lasts six to nine months

CONS

- can be expensive over a three-to-five year period
- maintenance required every five to nine months
- can be temporarily lumpy or uneven
- skin can appear uneven or bruised immediately after injections
- gradually deflates

fect or are younger, use the midweight versions of the fillers, Restylane and Juvederm. Regardless of which you choose, you should weigh the pros and cons for using a hyaluronic-acid filler for cheekbone definition.

Sculptra.   In expert hands, this can give a very smooth, natural contour. It builds up your skin naturally by increasing your own collagen.

Radiesse.   Radiesse is a filler composed of calcium hydroxylapatite crystals, a naturally occurring substance similar to cartilage. Thin connective tissue forms around the crystals once they are injected, anchoring the filler in place, while it is slowly absorbed by the body. However, there have been reports of inflamed bumps that do not resolve quickly. Usually one or two syringes are used in each cheek, resulting in an immediate and long-lasting correction that can last about twelve to eighteen months. But longevity can be unpredictable. I recommend waiting on this product until more long-term safety information and comparison studies with other fillers are available.

SCULPTRA

PROS

- longer-term results after the initial series, meaning less maintenance later
- one treatment every twelve-to-eighteen months
- stays more even throughout the entire year (doesn't "deflate" as much)
- improves skin texture and color by building collagen

PROS

- more expensive up front: initial series can run two thousand (cheekbones) to six thousand dollars, depending on age and how much filling is needed
- can be temporarily lumpy or uneven
- takes about six months to achieve the desired result

Filler safety.   Neither Sculptra nor Radiesse has as good a safety profile as that of Restylane or Juvederm. If Radiesse is injected only in the areas it is intended for (never lips), and the procedure is expertly done, it may be a good choice for you. It is not as forgiving as Juvederm, Restylane, or even Sculptra, in that any lumps that might form are not as easy to get rid of.

Remember, Juvederm and Restylane have the best safety profile of any injectable. If any bumps form, they can be quickly dissolved by injecting a few drops of hyalurondiase, an enzyme that dissolves hyaluronic acid. If you have a history of allergies or have experienced reactions to a wide variety of products, then definitely opt for the Juvederm and Restylane family of hyaluronic-acid products.

Cheek implants.   This is a plastic surgery procedure and, as with any plastic surgery, there are risks of bleeding, infection, scarring, and the anesthesia itself carries a risk. Implants are plastic so there can be a hard line of demarcation between the implant and normal tissue—occasionally even a visible ridge. These are best for posttrauma facial reconstruction.

REAL-WORLD ADVICE

I'm thirty-nine, and my cheekbones seem less defined now. What would you recommend?   I would recommend Juvederm Ultra Plus or Perlane. Injecting one or two syringes every nine or even twelve months would probably be enough at your age. I think it would be more cost effective than Sculptra as long as you don't have much sagging at the jawline.

I'm fifty-five, fairly thin, and would like to have my cheekbones look less bony and my cheeks look less hollow. What would you recommend? Without seeing you it's a little difficult, but I would probably recommend Sculptra. My guess is that at fifty-five you need the volume replaced in your entire cheek area, not just over your cheekbones. That way, you can fill the hollow areas, get a nice long-lasting result, and soften your cheekbone contour a bit.

I'm forty-seven and have never had much in the way of cheekbones. Is there some way to try one of these and see if I like the effect?   Yes, absolutely, but definitely go with the shorter-acting filler like Restylane/Juvederm. That way, if you don't like it, it would only last four to six months. You can always change to Juvederm Ultra Plus, Perlane, or Sculptra later if you want a longer-lasting result.

WRINKLES ON THE CHEEKS

Problem: Wrinkles on the cheek
Best Solutions: Lasers or peels

Lasers are best for wrinkles on the cheeks and work synergistically with Thermage and fillers. Please remember that excellent laser centers across the country will often use different lasers to get to the same end result. The exact laser or combination of lasers is less important than the experience, knowledge, and skill of the dermatologist using the laser or supervising the treatments. There are three main types of laser systems for wrinkles.

Lasers

Resurfacing lasers.   Common ones are the carbon-dioxide or erbium lasers. These lasers work by taking a thin, controlled layer off the entire surface of the skin. Healing time is seven to fourteen days with pinkness or red often remaining for several months. Usually one to two treatments are needed.

Fractional resurfacing lasers.   Common ones are the Fraxel, Affirm, Lux 1540, and the Active-Fx. So far the most studied and most useful of these is the Fraxel laser. These lasers work by damaging the skin and allowing it to heal with new collagen, like aerating your lawn. This pixel-like pattern can be microscopic (like the Fraxel) or larger (the Active-Fx). For the Fraxel treatment, healing time is minimal and most normal activities can be resumed within a day or two. Some brown or red discoloration is possible afterwards for a month or two. Treatments are usually done in a series of two to four.

Collagen-building lasers.   CoolTouch, Smoothbeam, or Aramis. These "long-wave" lasers work by selectively building the collagen to fill in the wrinkles. With most of these lasers, you could back to work with makeup on immediately but results are not as dramatic. Better for younger patients with minimal wrinkling. Usually done in a series of treatments.

Choosing a Treatment

Which treatment you choose for this area will depend on how deep the wrinkles are and how damaged your skin really is.

For minimal or shallow wrinkles.   You might think about using the collagen-building lasers, because there is no downtime. A series of five treatments over four to six months should give you some visible improvement. A word of caution: these lasers (except the Aramis) are quite uncomfortable and require prenumbing cream. You could also consider two or three treatments with a fractional laser.

For moderate or severe wrinkles.   For these, if you really cannot afford *any* redness or downtime then opt for a longer series (six to ten) with the collagen-building lasers. Otherwise, fractional lasers like the Fraxel, are better for moderate wrinkles and resurfacing lasers are more effective for deep wrinkles.

Peels.   Chemical peels, such as a TCA, or tricholoracetic acid peel, can be helpful for mild to moderate wrinkles on the cheeks. A full-face peel should be done, though, to avoid the peeled skin being a different texture or color. I never recommend phenol peels because they leave the skin completely white no matter what your original skin type is, without any melanin protection at all, and it looks very unnatural.

REAL-WORLD ADVICE

Why are there so many options for wrinkles on the cheeks?   The reason, unfortunately, is that no single treatment is really perfect. The resurfacing lasers need to be passed over the entire face to get even color and texture, but have too many risks and have too much downtime for many to consider. The other options, like the Fraxel or collagen-building lasers, and peels, will improve but not remove all the wrinkles. I generally tell my patients to expect between 40 and 80 percent improvement depending on their skin and on the technology used, the skill of the cosmetic dermatologist, and the number of treatments done. Combinations of all of the above can be used.

I have wrinkles on my upper cheeks, extending from my crow's feet down onto the cheek. What would be the best option for me?   I would recommend a fractional laser like the Fraxel or collagen-building lasers like the Smoothbeam or Cooltouch. And, a little Botox to relax the muscles in the crow's foot area. You might also need a little volume replacement with Sculptra or Juvederm Ultra Plus to support the upper cheek underneath the wrinkles.

I have deep wrinkles all over my cheeks. What should I do?   If you don't mind hiding out at home for ten to fourteen days, a carbon-dioxide or deep erbium laser resurfacing will give you the best and fastest results. For those of us who just can't get the time off, then I'd recommend a series of treatments (usually four to five) with the Fraxel laser. Then, add volume back with Sculptra, if you are too hollow.

I have wrinkles mostly on my lower cheeks. What would you recommend?   First look to see if the wrinkles on your lower cheek are caused by loss of volume in the upper cheek. If they are, replace the volume first and then go after the wrinkles with the devices mentioned above. Peels are always an option, and may be less expensive.

SLEEP LINES

These are those odd wrinkles that show up, seemingly overnight, on some women. Sleep lines usually occur on one side of the face only and are often vertical, rather than horizontal. They can be found anywhere and are caused by pressing our faces into our pillows at night in one position. If you think that odd line you are seeing might be a sleep line, try switching your pillow to something softer, or switching your sleeping position and see if that doesn't make it better. As we get older, these sleep lines can become permanent. They can be injected with CosmoPlast or a little Restylane to fill them back out again.

HOW WEIGHT CHANGES AFFECT THE CHEEKS

When I was pregnant, my cheeks seemed to get rounder and rounder with every pound I gained. I remember looking in the mirror one day and almost not recognizing myself. My cheekbones seemed to have disappeared. I think most, if not all of us, have had an experience like this where we've gained weight and the fat pads in our cheeks have gained weight, too. In addition to rounding out our faces, those fat pads in our cheeks also help to fill out any wrinkles.

I joked with one of my patients recently, who happened to have a fairly low body weight, that if she would just gain twenty or thirty pounds, probably all of those wrinkles in her cheeks would go away. Conversely, if you lose twenty or thirty pounds, you will notice more wrinkling through the cheek area, especially if you're in your forties or fifties, because you don't have the same elasticity and fat pads that you did in your twenties. Your skin acts like a balloon going up and down.

Sometimes patients ask me if the fact that they have gained and lost weight a number of times will have a permanent effect on their faces. When you are young, your skin has the most elasticity it will ever have; weight fluctuations don't affect the skin quite so much because the skin just bounces back. As you get older and you lose some of that elasticity, however, changes in weight may create some permanent sagging through the cheek area. It's simply harder for the skin to bounce back.

REAL-WORLD ADVICE

I've made a commitment to lose thirty pounds over the next year or two. Should I wait to get Thermage until I've lost the weight if my face needs a little bit of tightening? That depends on time and money. If your budget is very tight, I would vote for waiting until you are within ten or so pounds of your target weight to have the Thermage done. The doctor or nurse will be able to see better which areas to concentrate on. If money isn't as much of an issue, then you could have one treatment now and see some tightening, and then, in a year, repeat the procedure a second time to achieve the look you want.

I'm training for a triathlon and my total body fat is at an all-time low. I feel like I'm looking really gaunt. Would you recommend Sculptra or some other filler at this point?   If you tend to stay at a low body weight, then I don't think the timing matters so much. If your weight tends to go up five or ten pounds between competitions, then I would recommend you wait until you are done with the triathlon and your weight has stabilized before you decide if you want a series of Sculptra treatments.

FACELIFTS: A LAST RESORT

I still do refer some of my patients for facelifts if I think that the nonsurgical options will not provide enough tightening or be dramatic enough for their goals. I think a facelift, if it's done *once,* and isn't too tight, can be lovely for the right person. Multiple facelifts look pulled and unnatural most of the time. And, paradoxically, I don't think some women (or men) look younger after multiple facelifts. Most look their age, just stretched. And too much stretching looks unnatural. Nor do facelifts improve the skin color or texture itself. The stretching will reduce some wrinkles, yes. But if your skin is dry and blotchy or you have upper lip lines, a facelift won't help that.

If you decide to go the facelift route, do your research very carefully. Talk to at least two surgeons, and if they substantially disagree with each other in their approaches, talk to a third. Take your time. This is one surgery where making hasty decisions, or going solely by price, is a huge mistake. Generally speaking, the better surgeons are higher priced because they are more in demand and have more experience.

On average, facelifts last from five to fifteen years. If you do decide on a facelift, consider using Thermage every one to two years after that to maintain and extend the results.

THE BOTTOM LINE

- Use that sunscreen!
- If your cheeks need tightening, use Thermage or the Titan laser.
- If your cheeks need volume, use Sculptra, Juvederm or Restylane, or fat.
- If your cheekbones need definition, use Sculptra, Juvederm, or Restylane.
- To treat mild wrinkles on the cheek, use collagen-building laser treatments or a peel.
- Moderate to severe wrinkles in the cheek area require fractional resurfacing, traditional resurfacing, or a deeper peel.

YOUR JAWLINE AND CHIN

*The future belongs to those who believe
in the beauty of their dreams.*
—Eleanor Roosevelt

Women want a smooth jawline without jowls, lumps, bumps, or an S-shaped curve to it. All sorts of jaw shapes can be beautiful. I have patients who are beautiful with rounded jaws, narrow jaws, and square jaws. Here's what I hear:

- "I feel like I'm starting to sag here" (pointing to the jawbone).
- "Can you get rid of these jowls?"
- "I wish I could just pull everything up" (pulling up at the hairline).

A SAGGING JAWLINE

Problem: Mild to moderate loose skin along the jawline and chin
Best Solution: Nonsurgical skin tightening with Thermage

The best time to start treatments is when you see the very first signs of sagging—usually in the early- to midforties. It's easier to prevent and correct mild sagging than it is to correct a lot of sagging (usually in the late fifties and beyond).

We can often tell what we are headed for just by looking at our mothers. For example, my mother has terrible leg veins, and I could tell even in my early twenties that if I wanted to avoid her veins, I was going to have to start early with maintenance. I used support hose when pregnant and leg vein injections every three to four years starting in my midtwenties. The strategy of starting early and preventive maintenance has worked for me and will work for you, too.

As for fixing the things we don't like, I'm grateful that we have so many more options now. Most of this technology didn't even exist fifteen years ago.

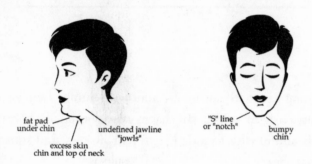

MAKE A LIST OF WHAT'S BOTHERING YOU

- jawline not defined
- excess skin under the chin
- excess skin at the top of the neck
- an S-shaped line with a notch just below the corner of the mouth
- bumpy chin

So what is the best nonsurgical option if you're in your forties or fifties and have some loose skin along the jawline? If the amount of loose skin is minimal to moderate, then Thermage, the skin-tightening system through radiofrequency, is still the best non-surgical solution. You may have also heard of Titan, a laser-based system that claims skin tightening effects similar to Thermage. Most of my colleagues who have used this, however, have not been impressed with the early Titan system. That said, the Titan has improved in the last few years. A series of three Titan treatments may now have similar effects to one Thermage. The Titan is also more painful than the third-generation Thermage. If you are sixty or over and have quite a bit of sagging, then surgery may, unfortunately, still be your best option.

Is Thermage painful?   A little history is helpful here because the Thermage (third generation) that dermatologists now use is vastly different from the Thermage of four or five years ago. The original (first generation) Thermage was overhyped by the media and some doctors with promotions like a "lunchtime lift" or before-and-after photos that were too good to be true. The treatments were painful without sedation (we sedated everyone in our office), and the results were inconsistent. Even worse, some doctors didn't follow the published protocols and turned the energy up too high causing an occasional depression in the skin.

Then came the second generation Thermage. This was still painful (our office still sedated everyone). But it worked more consistently because the handpiece used on the skin was equipped with a larger tip size (the tip is the part that delivers sound energy to the skin) and delivered more pulses per tip.

With the third generation of tips, the treatments have vastly improved. Thermage doubled the tip size, gave doctors many options for numbers of pulses in the tips (we usually use six hundred to eight hundred pulses for the full face), and added a cooling element to the tip so there is no pain. The treatment is now comfortable without sedation. I know from personal experience because I've had a treatment with each of the three generations of tips. What's more, all of our recent patients have had Thermage treatments without any medication whatsoever and were able to go back to their jobs and lives right away.

Thermage results.   The success of the procedure has also improved significantly, again due to the larger tip size and greater number of total pulse options. As mentioned earlier, when fifty-seven hundred patients who used the newer "multipass" version were surveyed at multiple clinics, 87 percent observed some immediate tightening while 92 percent had tightening six months after treatment. Ninety-four percent found that the treatment results met their expectations. This is consistent with the experience we've had at our clinic in Seattle.

As for safety, radiofrequency energy has been used in operating rooms all over the country for more than twenty-five years. The Thermage device is FDA approved. Studies showed a very small incidence of minor and temporary side effects.

The areas that Thermage improves.   The whole face and jawline can be treated to tighten the cheeks, reduce the fold between the nose and the mouth (nasolabial fold), and to tighten and lift the jowls. Thermage can also be performed on the forehead to lift the eyebrows and

---

QUESTIONS TO ASK WHEN GETTING INFORMATION ABOUT THERMAGE

- Who does it in the office? (You want a doctor, PA-C, or RN.)
- How many pulses are being used for a full face? (Five hundred to eight hundred is good.)
- Does the full face include under the chin? (It should.)
- How much time is booked for the entire procedure? (It should be 60–120 minutes.)
- Can the eyelids be done at the same time (Yes, they can.)

make the eyes look more open (see chapter 3), and it can be helpful on the neck if there isn't too much loose skin. Success at sites on the rest of the body has not been as consistent but it is also used to tighten the abdominal skin, the front of the thighs and upper arms. There is a new tip for body work which works more deeply and may be better.

You can go right back to work.   You will notice some immediate tightening of the skin, and a bit of puffiness (which disappears in one to three days and is unnoticeable to anyone else), immediately after the procedure, but there should be no bruising of any kind. Any pinkness generally disappears within several hours. With Thermage, you can put your makeup on and go right back to work (I've done this myself). All together, it takes about one to two hours to complete the process, and you are back on your way. You may return to your normal activities immediately after the Thermage treatment.

Long-lasting effects.   Treatment results (increased collagen) have been observed to last for at least two years. Thermage is not a surgical facelift, so you will not see a dramatic change in your face. As with virtually all skin restorative techniques, including surgical facelifts, the original aging symptoms slowly return as the aging and sun damage process continue. There are no studies on how often to repeat Thermage, but generally every one to two years should be sufficient.

Cost.   The cost for this procedure, depending on where you live, is usually somewhere from twenty-five hundred to four thousand dollars. Again, this procedure is best for those with mild to moderate sagging.

REAL-WORLD ADVICE

I have an event in two months. When would be the best time to do Thermage?   Remember that even though you will see a little bit of tightening right away with Thermage, most tightening occurs gradually over a period of four to six months. If your event is in two months, you'll see only a little improvement prior to the event.

I have a really busy social life and cannot afford any downtime at all. Would Thermage work for me?   Yes. Thermage is perfect for someone like you because you can have your treatment and walk right back out with no marks on your face. There is a very slight puffiness for a day or two that no one but you will notice, and that's it.

I know I'm not a good Thermage candidate, but I absolutely don't want surgery. Would I get at least some result?   Some of my patients don't want to undertake the risks, or have medical conditions that won't allow elective surgeries. You can certainly do two or three Thermage treatments approximately six months apart. With a combination of several Thermages and a series of Sculptra treatments, you can get a "non-surgical facelift" effect but it will not be as dramatic as a surgical facelift.

Is there anyone who shouldn't do Thermage?   Anyone who has a pacemaker or internal cardiac defibrillator, active skin infections in the treated area, or is pregnant should not have this procedure. Don't do Thermage over areas where you have a permanent fill like Artefill or silicone, because we don't know if they interact. Use caution and discuss with your doctor if you've had prior Sculptra treatments. Thermage is fine over Restylane and Juvederm.

Does Thermage work for the neck?   When I refer to Thermage on the neck, I mean the actual neck skin, not the loose skin just under the chin (some people get confused about this). I've not been impressed with Thermage on neck skin. I'm not sure why it isn't as successful there. Maybe because the skin is so much thinner than on the face, a special tip needs to be devised for the thinner neck skin.

I had a Thermage done and really didn't see much change. Why? There could be several reasons: (1)Enough pulses might not have been put in for your skin. We routinely use six hundred to eight hundred pulses in my office and occasionally even more if someone has a large face or a lot of laxity. (2)Technique is important with Thermage. It is important that the nurse or doctor pull in the correct directions while doing Thermage and that they do several full passes and even do five or six or seven passes with what is called the vector method. (3)There is a chance that you just don't do well with

Thermage. I have very few patients, but a few, who fall in that category. (4) You might be expecting too much.

FULL-FLEDGED JOWLS

Problem: A lot of sagging and loose skin along the jaw line
Best Solution: Plastic surgery

One of my patients once pointed to her jowls and told me she felt like a bulldog. We both laughed, but I know this is not a good feeling. This is one area where surgery really is the best option and here's why. If you really have full-fledged jowls, nonsurgical techniques cannot tighten enough to make it worth spending the money on them.

If you have a lot of loose skin at your jawline or at the upper part of your neck, you could do ten Thermages and it still wouldn't make a significant difference. Also, you want to be cost effective with your money, and if you spend $10,000 on Thermage and Sculptra and still have too much skin there, you will be disappointed and be out a lot of money. It would be far better to take fifteen to twenty-five thousand dollars (depending on which region you live in) and get a really great result. The recovery time for this kind of surgery is usually two to four weeks, with some bruising lasting longer than that and some swelling often lasting for three to six weeks. But usually, you can be back to your normal activities within weeks with

WHAT CAUSES JOWLS?

- sun damage to the cheek area
- loss of fat pads with shrinkage of the cheeks and chin
- loss of elasticity
- genes
- loss of bone with aging

makeup. Then, you can maintain the area with Thermage, usually having one every other year or perhaps even every year if needed.

REAL-WORLD ADVICE

I have a medical condition that makes it impossible for me to have any elective surgery—it's too risky. Please just give me everything I can do nonsurgically to improve this area. I'm not trying to look perfect.   Usually a combination of several Thermages, Fraxel lasers, and Sculptra or the longer-lasting Juvederm or Restylane is optimal. You will need a good cosmetic dermatologist to help you with the sequence and timing of it all. And plan on needing approximately a year to complete everything.

I'm on a budget and getting Thermage done is really a financial stretch for me. I'm scared that I won't get the results but will have spent the money.   First, make sure that you are thinking about Thermage for the right reasons. If you're considering it because you need a little bit of tightening on your cheek area and along the jawline, but you're not expecting any improvement in either redness or brown spots, then it sounds like you're on the right track. Also think about whether there are other, less expensive things that would make a difference in your appearance for less money—for example, treatment of red blood vessels on your cheeks or age or brown spots. If texture is a problem, maybe some peels, which can range between one hundred to two hundred each, would give you a boost without costing as much money.

"NOTCHING" ALONG THE JAWLINE

Problem: Jawline starts to have an S shape
Best Solution: Restylane, Juvederm, or Sculptra

You're probably wondering what I'm talking about. Some people get two little indentations that occur on the jawline directly below the outside corners of their mouth such that the contour of the jaw is no longer smooth and looks more like a modified S shape. Medically this is called the prejowl sulcus. This notch is caused by different things. For example, excess skin along the jawbone will emphasize that little indentation, shrinking of the fat pad in the chin area will cause the indentation, and sometimes overactivity of the muscle that holds down the corners of the mouth, called the depressor anguli oris (DAO) muscle, worsens notching.

A combination of treatments here is usually best, but in your particular situation, one alone might do the trick.

If the problem is more that the chin area itself is thinning or that the DAO muscle (the muscle that pulls the corners of the mouth down) is too active, then filling the area with Juvederm or Restylane would be best. A drop of Botox here may also help.

If the notching is being caused by an S shape due to sagging skin on the lateral part of the jaw or the outside part of the jawline, then Thermage or longer-acting fillers to bring the excess skin up or a combination of the two of them would be the best.

REAL-WORLD ADVICE

I want the creases from my nose to my mouth and my mouth to my chin filled in a bit. Can the notch be done at the same time?   Yes, with Restylane or Juvederm. In fact, it's best to fill both of those areas and that indented area at the sides of the chin at the same time so you have a smooth jaw contour.

I'm thirty-nine and my only problem along my jawline is that the indentation is starting. What would be best for this?   I would recommend a half or full syringe of Restylane or Juvederm. If you're young and don't have other creases that you are trying to fill in, then that should be enough to do that area and not too expensive.

If I have that notching at my jawline and a lot of sagging through my cheek area. Which filler would be best for me?   Sculptra or perhaps the thicker Perlane or Juvederm Ultra Plus would be best in your situation. You will want a very long-lasting, low-maintenance filler that will give you a lot of volume. The thicker Juvederm Ultra Plus and Perlane fill well but it takes more filler for the cheeks, and is more expensive than Sculptra over several years. They also don't last as long, and you won't get the youthful glow that you will with Sculptra due to the collagen growth that Sculptra stimulates. While Sculptra has full approval in the European Union and Canada, it has limited FDA approval in the United States (HIV only—other uses are "off-label"). Full approval is expected in 2008.

COBBLESTONE CHIN

Problem: Bumpy skin on the chin
Best Solution: Botox

One of my patients described this as cellulite of the chin—that bumpy, lumpy skin in the chin area that develops over time. I've always called it cobblestone chin. When I go to the European conference on aging skin, the French call it *peau d'orange.* They think it looks like the skin of an orange. Some women never develop this and, like many things about skin, there probably is a genetic component to it.

The easiest way to remedy this is just a couple of very small drops of Botox in the chin area. This relaxes the muscle just enough that it doesn't cause the dimpling. When I say drops, I literally mean drops. I do this as an adjunct to treating other areas on the face. This usually works so well that there is no need for a filler, but some excellent dermatologists use a little Restylane or CosmoPlast to fill in some of the depressed areas.

THE RECEDING CHIN

Problem: Chin recedes
Best Solution: Augmentation with Juvederm or Restylane

It used to be the only way to remedy a receding chin was with a chin implant. If your chin is receding dramatically, it may be that you're also having trouble with your bite. Be sure to get an evaluation by a good dentist or an oral surgeon prior to any procedure, because your jawbone itself may need to be realigned. Imagine getting a chin implant, only to find out you needed a more extensive surgery to correct serious bite problems or TMJ (temporal mandibular joint) problems!

Even assuming that there are no serious dental or TMJ issues, I'm still not a fan of chin implants. Generally made of plastic, they come with the same complications all surgeries do. They can also move and get infected. I have one patient in whom I can see a clear drop off at the sides of the implant on her chin as she's gotten older, and some of the skin around the implant has thinned a little bit. Having said that, I do know some patients who are happy with them.

A nonsurgical alternative would be to use one of the longer-lasting, thicker, higher-molecular-weight fillers such as Juvederm Ultra Plus. You'd be surprised at how much you can augment and contour the chin area with a syringe. These fillers have even been used for contouring noses and in some cases have eliminated the need for surgical correction of some nose defects. Try the temporary (lasting six to twelve months) filler first to see how it looks. If it works, then you might save yourself the surgery. If not, you always have the option of a chin implant later.

THE BOTTOM LINE

Try that maneuver again—the one where you pull up the front of your ears and watch under your chin and the neck area. All of these areas are connected as one piece of skin, so if your cheeks are sagging, your jawline will sag. If your jawline sags, it will cause sagging in the neck. Conversely, if you improve any of these areas, all of them will improve some.

- For mild to moderate sagging along the jawline, try Thermage, Sculptra, or both. It's safer to do the Thermage before the Sculptra.
- For full-fledged jowls, surgery is your best option.
- For a bumpy chin, try a few drops of Botox.
- If you have a notch at the jawline just under the corners of the mouth, fill with Restylane or Juvederm.
- And for a receding chin, try Juvederm UltraPlus first, and then consider a surgical implant. Get an oral surgery evaluation first.

YOUR NECK AND CHEST

To me, fair friend, you can never be old. For as you were when first your eye I eyed, such seems your beauty still.
—William Shakespeare, "Sonnet 104"

Do our feelings about our necks really encapsulate our feelings about aging? Maybe so. And truthfully, wrinkles on the neck are one of the hardest areas to improve nonsurgically. But hope is on the horizon. Sometimes new technology really does make a difference.

Here are the main questions I hear about the neck and chest:

- "How can I get the skin on my face, neck, and chest to match?"
- "What products should I use on my neck and chest?"
- "What can I do about those horizontal 'necklace' lines on my neck?"
- "My neck and chest are blotchy."
- "My chest is wrinkly and sun damaged."

WHICH PRODUCTS ARE BEST ON THE NECK AND CHEST

Problem: Protecting the more delicate skin on the neck and chest
Best Solution: Sunscreens and antioxidants

MAKE A LIST OF WHAT'S BOTHERING YOU

- neck too crepey
- horizontal "necklace" lines
- neck discolored—red or brown and blotchy
- prominent upper-neck vertical bands that stick out
- wrinkled and leathery chest
- blotchy chest

Taking Care of the Skin on Your Neck and Chest

This is my golden rule number one. Put the same sunscreen on your neck and chest as you do on your face—and on the backs of your hands too. This may sound obvious, but it's amazing how many of us don't do it—including myself. When I was in my midtwenties, I started sunscreening my face regularly. But I didn't start covering my neck and chest until five years later. It suddenly dawned on me one morning that I was starting to see sun damage on these areas and that I needed to protect all three.

So, some tips for keeping your neck and chest looking their best:

- Apply sunscreen to your neck, chest, and face every morning.
- Use a good moisturizer under your sunscreen in the morning and at night. Your neck, especially, has very few oil glands.
- Some products that are fine on your face will be irritating on your neck/chest area—usually the neck—because your skin is very thin there. You may need to adjust the frequency or strength of vitamin-A creams like Renova or antioxidant creams to the neck and chest area to avoid irritation. First try using them every other night instead or dilute them with your moisturizer. Then, if still irritated, try twice a week.

- If your neck or chest gets irritated from a product, stop the product, use over-the-counter hydrocortisone cream 0.5 percent or 1.0 percent for a few days with lots of moisturizer—three or four times a day. The irritation should calm down in a few days. If it doesn't, see your dermatologist.

Repairing the neck and chest skin with products.   Many of my patients ask me if it's possible to repair sun damage on the neck and chest with creams. I would say the answer is a very limited yes. Good products can help with very fine lines and give a slight improvement in texture and some color problems, but if there is even minimal sun damage, you'll probably need repair work with lasers or peels.

What sort of products should you use? The neck and chest area have far fewer oil glands than your face. You will want a richer, heavier moisturizer for this area unless you have acne on the chest. We've already covered good moisturizers in chapter 1, but here are some effective ones (that aren't too expensive) to use on this particular area:

- Bobbi Brown Hydrating Face Cream—for normal to dry skin (available at department stores)
- Cetaphil Moisturizing Cream—for dry, sensitive skin (available at your drugstore)
- La Mer—for dry skin (available at department stores, but expensive)
- Neutrogena Healthy Skin Lotion—for normal to dry skin (available at your drugstore)
- Olay Total Restoration Lotion—for normal to dry skin (available at your drugstore)
- MD Forte Replenish Hydrating Cream—for normal to dry skin (available online and at dermatologists' offices)

For sunscreens, the more expensive sunscreens really are better. This is because they contain higher amounts of the ingredients that block UVA as well as UVB. Many of the drugstore sunscreens that say "broad spectrum" have very little UVA coverage (think zinc, titanium, or mexoryl) compared to the more expensive brands.

Once you have your sunscreens and moisturizers, try adding an antioxidant. This will help prevent sun damage and possibly aid the skin with its own repair process. Try Prevage (idebenone) or the Cellex-C Vitamin C complex. You may need to use less if your neck gets irritated. Or try applying just two to three times per week.

For sunscreen on the neck and chest, I recommend either the Skin-Medica Environment Defense Sunscreen SPF 30, which contains 9 percent zinc in addition to other active ingredients, or Colorescience Sunforgetable SPF 30. Another good one is La Roche-Posay Anthelios, which has a combination of both chemical and physical UVA blockers. Both of these you will need to either get online or in a dermatologist's office.

For creams that help repair neck and chest skin, work with a dermatologist. The best ones, like the vitamin-A cousins (Renova, Tazorac, Retin-A, Retinol, etc.), repair damage by increasing collagen production, normalizing damaged cells, and increasing healthy cell activity. The products will need to be adjusted for your skin and can cause redness and irritation if you don't know how to use them correctly. Again, antioxidant products, such as the vitamin-C serums or idebenone, work more to prevent damage in the first place.

SKIN-TIGHTENING CREAMS FOR THE NECK— DO THEY WORK?

- No. There's nothing available in a jar or bottle that can tighten, despite the marketing claims.
- A good moisturizer and sunscreen are still the best products to start with.

REAL-WORLD ADVICE

I've had several bad sunburns on my chest. Can I repair this?   Yes. The first thing to do is to protect the area with clothing and quality sunscreens like the ones mentioned above. After protecting the area, consider investing in Fraxel or IPL laser treatments to repair the damage.

If you swim a lot or frequently visit vacation spots that are sunny, please ... please ... please get a surfer suit or rash guard (try *www.coolibar.com, sunprecautions.com*, surf shop web sites or Patagonia's Water Girl line). You won't believe how much wear and tear they'll save your skin in the water. I love to swim in Lake Washington in the summer in Seattle, and I always wear a surfer suit. It doesn't restrict your motion at all, and it's nice because you don't have to sunscreen so much of your body.

GETTING THE SKIN ON YOUR FACE, NECK, AND CHEST TO MATCH

Problem: That blotchy, red, and age-spot-speckled skin on the neck and chest
Best Solution: IPLs and lasers

TERMS YOU'LL WANT TO KNOW

- *platysmal band:* those stringy vertical bands on the upper neck that tend to stick out with age
- *submental:* under the chin, sometimes there is a fat pad here
- *clavicle:* the "collarbones"
- *thyroid:* the important gland at the base of the neck (you can't see it)
- *trachea:* "windpipe" that runs down the middle of the neck

How many times have you seen someone on the street or at a party whose facial skin looks quite good—maybe they've taken great care of it, or maybe they've had some work done, who knows. But, when you look at their neck and chest, you see sun-damaged, leathery skin. Let's face it, those mismatches look odd unless you plan to wear a turtleneck for the rest of your life.

Creams will go only so far to repair the neck and chest. Usually a series of laser treatments are needed to repair the skin and get it looking good again. You can then maintain the improvement with sunscreens and antioxidants and a maintenance laser treatment once or twice a year. Here's how to go about it.

IMPROVING THE SKIN ON YOUR NECK AND CHEST WITH LASERS

Two Different Approaches

There are two ways to approach improving the skin on the neck and chest, depending on your time and budget constraints. One approach is to say, "My face, neck, and chest are all really sun damaged, and I'd like to improve all of them at the same time." If that's the case, then you can try a series of Fraxel laser treatments (usually three to five) or IPL (intense pulsed light) photorejuvenation treatments (usually four to six). Use the Fraxel if you are blotchy but also have wrinkles or texture problems and the IPL if you are just blotchy.

As these are usually done about a month apart, it will take approximately six months to finish the course. Plan on each appointment taking about sixty to ninety minutes, with the cost ranging from eight hundred to fifteen hundred dollars (per treatment) for the face, neck, and chest. At the end of that time, though, your skin should look great.

But other patients, due to either time or budget issues or different levels of sun damage on their faces, necks, and chests, may want to proceed more gradually. They may opt to treat the face first over a period of six months or so, and then gradually, over the next couple of years, tackle the neck and chest. Or, they may focus on different areas. For example, just two of the three areas might be sun damaged.

The Best Lasers for the Neck and Chest

Among cosmetic dermatologists, there are several camps regarding what type of laser to use. One camp favors using lasers to treat the brown spots individually and then using a different laser to treat the red areas individually. The other camp (and this is the camp I'm in) likes to use IPLs (intense pulsed light devices, which are like close cousins to lasers) on the neck and chest. The IPLs do a better job (remember—doctor's offices have more powerful IPLs than spas), because you can treat both the brown spots and the red discoloration at the same time. In addition, photorejuvenation with the IPL should also give you some improvement in the texture of your skin through collagen rebuilding. But both will work, and the skill and experience of the doctor is more important than the exact laser or IPL system.

IPL-type lasers.   Here's how the IPL device for photorejuvenation works: The IPL light targets hemoglobin (the pigment inside red blood cells). The laser beam passes through the skin and is absorbed by the red color. This damages the vessel wall, and then the tiny, damaged red blood vessels are absorbed by the body and made less visible. The redness goes away! The same thing holds for the brown spots on your chest. These are made of melanin, and the IPL can target melanin to make the brown go away.

Studies have also shown that the laser light stimulates cells in the deeper layers of the skin that make collagen. After the light hits them, they begin to make new collagen over a period of many months. This often results in smoother skin with a slight decrease in fine lines. Don't try to use this process to remove crepey lines on the neck, however. IPLs really don't make a difference on wrinkles on the neck. They are specifically for redness and brown spots.

The average number of treatments you'll need to remove redness and dilated blood vessels effectively on the neck is three to six depending on the amount of sun damage you have. The neck and chest *can* take even more treatments than the face.

How are the laser treatments done?   When you come to a laser center, you will be shown to a "laser room." A nurse or technician will put special glasses or eyepads over your eyes to protect them. A cool gel is then placed on the skin being treated. The smooth glass surface of the handpiece is gently applied to your skin and pulses of light flash. You may feel a very slight sting, like the snapping of a small rubber band. At the end of the treatment, the nurse wipes off the gel, cleans the area with a warm cloth, and applies a moisturizer with sunscreen. If there is any mild swelling, you might be given a cold pack to apply for five or ten minutes. Most centers will let you reapply foundation or concealer immediately after a treatment. The treatment time varies depending on how large the treatment area is, but thirty to ninety minutes is typical.

Do the treatments hurt?   You may experience some mild discomfort during the treatments, but you'll be able to tolerate it pretty easily. The redder your neck is, the larger the target for the lasers, so the first one or two treatments are more uncomfortable than later treatments. As you get closer to resolution, though, the treatments become noticeably less uncomfortable. In some centers, you may be allowed to use a topical numbing cream. If your laser treatments seem uncomfortable, also try taking some Tylenol the night before and the morning of your treatment.

Try not to take aspirin, ibuprofen, or naprosyn (Aleve) the week prior to your treatment, because they will make you more likely to bruise (don't forget that Excedrin contains aspirin). If you are taking those medications for medical reasons, ask your primary care doctor first to make sure it's okay to stop them for a week.

As far as exercise goes, you may be asked to refrain from vigorous exercise or yoga for several days after the treatment. Stay out of the sun! If you must go out in it, use good sunscreen and a hat. You may feel a slight burning sensation right after the treatment or even overnight and you may have mild to moderate puffiness for a day or two.

Complications are rare, but if you develop any blistering or crusting, be sure to call your dermatologist to find out how she would like you to care for the area. This is superficial and generally doesn't result in any long-term problems, but your doctor may have a special regimen for treatment of those areas. Permanent scarring is very, very rare so long as you follow all of the posttreatment instructions that are given to you, call with any problems, and go to a reputable center.

Fractional-resurfacing lasers.   These lasers have become available in the past few years and are very promising in improving blotchy, crinkly, or sun-damaged skin on the neck and chest. The best studied and most used of these lasers is the Fraxel. It does not work well for redness, however, just brown pigment, wrinkles, and other texture problems.

For a Fraxel laser treatment, a patient's experience is different from that with the IPLs. You will be asked to arrive at your laser center about an hour to an hour and a half before your treatment actually starts. After you are put in a room, makeup removed, and a headband or cap put on to protect your hair, a thick numbing ointment will be applied all over your face and into your hairline. Be sure to tell your doctor or nurse if you have had any problems with numbing creams or shots at the dentist in the past. For a video clip see www.skintour.com.

After you numb for about an hour, the numbing gel will be removed. With first-generation Fraxel I, a blue dye is then applied. With the newer Fraxel II, the dye is not necessary. You'll be taken to the laser room, made comfortable, and a thin layer of gel will be applied to help the laser rollers slide evenly over the face. The treatment takes about an hour and feels a little like a "pins and needles" sensation.

When you leave, you will be red, but the redness fades gradually over one to three days turning into a slight bronzing (it looks like a tan) that then takes two to four weeks to resolve. Makeup can be worn, and other people usually don't notice anything except for the first few days. There are subtle texture changes which take two to four weeks to resolve, but they can only be felt, not seen.

There are other competing devices in this category, including the Affirm, the Active FX, and the Lux1540. The problem is that they haven't been used as long as the Fraxel to know whether they get consistently good results over a wide variety of patients. I'd recommend avoiding these lasers for the next year or two unless you live near a large center with doctors with extensive laser experience. Until we know their potential complications and they have proved themselves to give cost-effective and consistent results, caution is advised.

Photodynamic or Blu-U treatments.   You may have read about Blu-U or photodynamic laser treatments for sun damaged skin. This is another twist on treating the face, neck, or chest areas with an IPL.

With the Blu-U, a nurse or technician will pretreat your skin with a clear liquid called ALA, and then perform a light laser treatment about an hour later. This gives good results, usually after two or three treatments. What's the catch? Why not use this all the time instead of a series of five IPLs? The Blu U, or photodynamic therapy, results in significantly more redness and peeling, which equals more downtime. Most of my patients hate downtime and would rather get the same result after five IPLs with no downtime than three Blu-Us with five to seven days of redness and peeling following each. But if you're wearing turtlenecks all winter long or downtime isn't an issue, then you might want to inquire about this. The cost of each treatment is more because the cost of the ALA is added in.

REAL-WORLD ADVICE

I have a high school reunion coming up. How far in advance should I plan to start laser treatments?   You'll want to begin laser treatments six to nine months ahead of your event. Six months would be fine if you have mild to moderate redness or blotchiness. Start nine months ahead for best results if it is severe, since you may need more than five treatments.

I had a series of laser treatments on my neck at a medi-spa, and I really didn't see any results. Is there anything else I can do?   Unfortunately, I think you may have just wasted your money. Some of the medi-spa "techs" are trained for only a day or two before being allowed to use laser equipment. Much of the time, they undertreat. Also, the lasers and IPLs that are sold to salons and medi-spas are not always as powerful as the models that are sold to doctors' offices. The medi-spa may have used a weaker laser or one that can't be customized to your skin. I would recommend approaching a reputable, established laser center, run by a dermatologist for a second opinion.

I started a series of laser treatments but found it so uncomfortable I just couldn't continue. What could be the problem?   It may just be that you are extremely red or brown and blotchy so there is a lot of target for the IPL or laser to hit. At our laser center, we will sometimes use numbing cream for the first couple of treatments if you are very red or have a lot of sun/age spots. You might ask if they use numbing cream in your laser center. Also, everyone's nerve endings are a little different. Some people have really sensitive nerve endings. If you are one of those people, you might want to let your doctor know. You can try taking Tylenol the night before and the morning of the treatment to lessen the discomfort.

My chest has mostly brown spots and just a few veins. Will photorejuvenation still be effective?   Yes, at excellent centers that use photorejuvenation frequently, different filters may be used to target the brown spots; the IPL should work very nicely. You could also consider the Fraxel laser. If the brown spots are really raised or you've had trouble with precancerous lesions, then you need to clear up all the precancerous spots first with your doctor and then remove any raised spots that are not precancerous— usually these are referred to as seborrheic keratoses (I call them barnacles). This can be done with liquid nitrogen or by several other methods. After the raised or crusty areas are removed, you can then tackle the brown and red flat blotches on your chest with photorejuvenation or the Fraxel.

My face is pretty sun damaged, but my neck and chest look pretty good. Do I still need to get these areas treated?   No. In that case, I would treat your face, but focus on prevention for your neck and chest. Start with sunscreens, moisturizers, and perhaps an antioxidant.

NECKLACE LINES

Problem: The sometimes-deep horizontal lines on the neck
Best Solutions: Botox and/or light resurfacing lasers like the Fraxel or erbium

Necklace lines are the horizontal lines going across the neck. Some of my patients have absolutely none of these as time goes on, although they may have other problems on their necks. In others, this starts very early. While the medical literature is not definitive on what causes these lines, it seems to be due to the action of muscles under the skin. That would explain why we see these even in very young people.

If these lines are starting to get deep and are bothering you, the best treatment is a little Botox. Treatment for this in my office usually costs about two hundred dollars. I just put a few drops of Botox about a centimeter apart all across the necklace lines. This helps quite a bit and, in conjunction with all the moisturizer and sun protection I know you are using already on your neck, this should make them look significantly better over time. Light resurfacing or fractional lasers may improve their appearance as well.

THE CORDS IN MY NECK STICK OUT

Problem: Prominent vertical bands that stick out at the upper part of the neck
Best Solutions: Botox or surgery

Botox in these bands is helpful if the bands aren't too loose. The Botox relaxes the bands (the platysma muscles) so that they tuck back up under the jawline better.

There are several different surgical approaches to this problem so if your bands are quite loose or visible, get a surgical consultation with a plastic surgeon.

MY NECK IS RED AND BLOTCHY

Problem: That blotchy, red discoloration on the neck
Best Solution: Pulsed dye or IPL lasers

The neck and chest are a bit different. Sun damage on the neck shows up as redness initially that starts to persist. By age forty or fifty, that redness can become a permanent, blotchy, red area. This is where the term *redneck* came from. Farmers, particularly, or people who worked outdoors for many hours, developed this pattern of red, blotchy sun damage on the sides and back of the neck.

Photorejuvenation (explained above) or a pulsed dye laser are the most effective treatment for blotchy reddening on the neck. Pulsed dye lasers have an advantage on the neck if redness is the primary problem (not brown discoloration). If your redness or blotchiness is extensive, you may need more than the usual five treatments in a series. And if you don't see improvement after three or even four treatments, don't give up. I've seen pretty dramatic improvement after the fourth or fifth treatment of a pulsed dye laser or photorejuvenation. IPLs also work well and are better if the discoloration is both brown and red.

There is no cream or lotion at the moment that can take this type of redness away for anything longer than a few hours. Some people have tried to use over-the-counter hydrocortisone on it. Hydrocortisone will temporarily make it look a bit better—as in a few hours—but in the long run, overusing cortisone creams may thin the skin and make the problem worse. Makeup on the neck is not a good option because it rubs off on all your clothing. Once you've spent the time and money to correct this problem, be sure you apply sunscreen to your neck consistently so you're not just wasting your money.

WRINKLES AND CREPEY SKIN ON THE NECK

Problem: Those tiny fine lines and slightly loose skin on the neck
Best Solution: Light resurfacing lasers like the erbium or Fraxel

Not too long ago, if you came into my office bothered by that slightly loose, crepey skin on your neck that almost all of us get as time goes on, I would have said there wasn't a great option for nonsurgical repair. I would have told you to save your money and consider surgery when it gets bad enough.

True, there has been the option of a conventional resurfacing laser like the erbium but unless the treatments were done perfectly, usually by a laser expert, they could leave the neck scarred and discolored because the skin is so thin and dry. It was too risky to recommend wholeheartedly.

But now, there is some data supporting the use of the Fraxel laser to improve the neck skin. To understand how fractional resurfacing works, think about pixels (or aerating your lawn). The laser sends tiny, microscopic beams that shoot all the way from the top of the skin way down into the dermis. Because roughly only 15 to 20 percent of the skin is being replaced at each treatment, the skin heals much more quickly than when treated with the traditional resurfacing lasers. Fractional resurfacing treatments are approximately a thousand dollars per treatment on the neck. Usually two to four treatments are needed.

Here's what I know *doesn't* work well for wrinkles on the neck so you won't waste your money:

- Photorejuvenation. It's great for color problems on the neck but not for wrinkles.
- Peels. Light peels don't have much effect. Medium peels done carefully in a series may be useful. Deep peels are not safe because there is too much risk of scarring. If you have a cosmetic dermatologist who performs a lot of medium-depth peels on the neck, you might get good results.
- Thermage. I love Thermage, for the right person, on the face. But we've tried many different protocols on the neck, without much result. Having said that, Thermage has just come out with a new

tip specifically designed for thinner-skinned areas, like the hands. This tip may prove to work well on the neck, but there's no data to support that yet.

- Carbon-dioxide resurfacing lasers. Unless your doctor is one of the top five laser surgeons in the nation, don't let anyone use a conventional carbon dioxide resurfacing laser on your neck. It's just too risky. You'll likely develop scarring and pigmentation problems. Erbium lasers can be better here, but only in expert hands. A new plasma resurfacing laser is available, but is quite new, expensive, and lacks data on results.

I THINK I NEED A NECK LIFT

A neck lift is really a facelift. When women talk about a neck lift, we are probably deceiving ourselves just a bit. To pull the neck tighter, the surgeon has to cut around the ears at least somewhat in order to take up excess skin.

Sometimes what's called a minilift can be done, which involves incisions just around the lower part of the ear rather than a full facelift, which often goes much higher, sometimes even into the temple area. Here's when to consider surgery:

- You have a lot of wrinkles and loose skin on the neck, such that nonsurgical treatments really just aren't going to help.
- You have the above plus sagging under the chin and at the jowls.
- The platysmal bands (I've heard these sometimes referred to as turkey wattles) are pretty loose and clearly a problem.

Here's what surgery won't do:

- It won't fix color problems—you need to do that with a laser.
- It won't fix growths—please get any of those checked first by your dermatologist to make sure they are not precancerous, and get them removed prior to your surgery.
- It won't make thin skin any thicker.

WRINKLES AND LINES ON THE CHEST

Wrinkles on the chest occur naturally over time as part of sun damage. But I also see some women over fifty who have very little sun damage but still develop these lines.

The lines are often most noticeable in the morning, especially if you happen to be a side sleeper. And if you look at your chest before and after sleeping, you may notice you're getting certain wrinkles across the chest area that correspond to your sleeping position. I, for one, have a hard time sleeping on my back, and I know that some of my chest lines in the morning come from sleeping on my side.

The best option for treating these lines is a fractional laser like the Fraxel or a fractionated erbium laser. Some expert injectors, mostly in Europe, are using Sculptra on the chest.

THE BOTTOM LINE

- Start with a good moisturizer and sunscreen.
- Get a medical exam first, please—if you have growths, have them checked before you do any cosmetic work to make sure they are not skin cancers. The chest is prone to skin cancers.
- Color problems on the neck and chest—photorejuvenation with IPL (intense pulsed light), a pulsed dye laser, or possibly fractional resurfacing laser (for brown spots) are the best.
- Necklace lines and vertical bands on the neck are best treated with Botox.
- If the wrinkles are mild to moderate on the neck, fractional resurfacing lasers are promising, but you may want to wait a year for more data to see what results you can expect. If the wrinkles on the neck are more severe, consider a "neck" lift surgery.
- Wrinkles on the chest can be treated with the Fraxel laser or other gentle fractional lasers.

PART THREE
FOCUS ON TEXTURE AND COLOR

9

BROWN SPOTS, AGE SPOTS, AND TOO RED?

Out, damn spot.
—MacBeth, William Shakespeare

One morning a fifty-four-year-old patient came to my office for a skin exam. The woman had virtually *no* sun damage. She didn't have one single brown or "age" spot on her entire body. Her face had a few dilated or broken blood vessels, but that was the extent of her sun damage.

I assumed that she'd spent the majority of her time out of the sun. So imagine my surprise when she said she'd been a long-distance runner and still ran five to ten miles outdoors four times a week. I was impressed. When I asked her how she managed to do so with so little sun damage, she explained she'd been slathering on sunscreen prior to any outdoor activity for her entire life, always wore a hat, and even sometimes ran in a moisture-wicking polypropylene turtleneck so that her neck would be covered.

Her skin is a wonderful testament to the fact that sun damage is preventable. Still, for most of us over the age of forty, some sun damage is evident. Almost all of us can point to a few brown spots, age spots, some redness, or dilated blood vessels (the redness could also be rosacea) that we don't like. Most of us haven't been as cautious as my patient when it comes to protecting our skin. And so, the question remains, in addition to being more proactive about protection in the future, what can we do to "reverse" the brown spots and redness that we see now?

BLOTCHINESS (BROWN SPOTS AND AGE SPOTS)

Age spots are sun damage! True, they come over time. And get worse the older we get. But they're mostly sun damage. One of my dermatology professors used to say with a smile, "If you don't believe me on this, just look at your grandmother's tushy." Her face and hands may have lots of brown spots where she's had sun exposure, but not her covered posterior.

Here are some common concerns from women in my office:

- "I was pregnant eight years ago, and the brown spots I got during the pregnancy have never gone away. What can I do?"
- "My mother has a lot of age spots, and now at age forty-five I am starting to get them too."
- "Are bleaching creams really okay to use?"
- "My physician recommended microdermabrasion to me for these spots. Will that work?"
- "I'm too young to get these liver spots on the backs of my hands!"

PREVENTING BROWN AND AGE SPOTS

Preventing sun damage is much easier than repairing it later. As discussed earlier, make sure your skin is protected from both UVB *and* UVA radiation. A surprising number of sunsceens don't protect against UVA. Here are the basics:

Make sure your sunscreen contains at least 5–10 percent of a good UVA blocker like zinc, titanium, or 3 percent Mexoryl. Remember that all sunscreens will block UVB, but UVA blocking is critical for prevention of brown spots and long-term sun damage. The SPFs on sunscreen refer only to UVB, not UVA.

Wear sunscreen on any exposed area every day. Think of the rug or couch or drapes in your living room that are exposed to light all day long. Think of the cracked and leathery texture of the sofa and the faded and weakened fibers in the drapes. That's what is happening to your skin! Make sure to reapply your sunscreen every couple of hours. Remember that covering up with clothing, particularly sun-protective clothing, is one of the best ways to avoid sun damage. See page 13 for important information on Vitamin D.

Is It Sun Damage, Melasma, or Something Else?

The first thing to do when trying to get rid of brown spots is to figure out the cause. If you can figure out what's causing your spots, it will be much easier to get an effective treatment. The main causes of brown blotches on your face are sun damage, melasma (large blotches caused by pregnancy, oral contraceptives, and postmenopausal hormone replacement therapy or HRT), picking, acne, and other skin diseases.

Some patients have multiple causes for their blotches. For example, one woman had some melasma left over from pregnancy years ago, brown spots from acne that left dark marks as it resolved, and brown spots from sun damage as well. Her situation is more complicated than most, but sometimes there's more than one thing going on. So, which do you have? Let's try to figure it out.

Brown Spots due to Sun Damage

Brown spots from sun damage usually show up first as what we call freckles. The medical name for freckles is *solar lentigos*. Freckles may look cute on a redheaded seven-year-old. But those freckles are sun damage.

If you are a redhead, of Celtic ancestry, or have lighter skin, you will be prone to brown spots from sun damage. They usually start up in childhood as small, discrete freckles and then over time coalesce into larger and larger brown blotches as more sun damage occurs. Or, if you're a more medium skin type, the brown spots will show up in later years. They're related to your cumulative sun exposure and to any sunburns you've had in the past.

African-Americans may have small, dark spots on the cheeks that look like freckles but are slightly raised. These are different in that they are usually inherited and not caused by sun damage. They are called *stucco keratoses* and can be removed.

Brown Spots due to Melasma

Melasma is the darkening of the skin, usually on the face, in irregular, often large splotches. It is caused by the hormones of pregnancy, birth control pills, or hormone replacement. Women of color are prone to melasma, and it is a significant problem for many. But people of any skin type can get melasma.

Some women will develop melasma along the sides of their face and their jawline, others mostly on the upper lip, and still others on the forehead. There's no predicting exactly where it will show up or who will be most susceptible.

Natural or prescribed estrogens (female hormones) plus sun are the main culprit. Melasma resulting from oral contraceptive use is particularly common. Gynecologists and family-practice doctors are the most likely physicians to be prescribing oral contraceptives, and many will warn their patients about this complication.

This is important because melasma, if caught early and treated aggressively, is much more likely to be limited or temporary. After it's gone on for many years, even if the offending agent is stopped, it sometimes becomes a long-term, even lifelong problem.

Melasma with pregnancy.   We most commonly think of melasma occurring in pregnancy. Almost all of us have had friends, whether they got pregnant at age twenty-five or at age forty-one, who have darkening on their faces during pregnancy. If melasma starts during a pregnancy, chances are good it will resolve itself after delivery. It may recur with subsequent pregnancies, though, particularly if you are pregnant during the summer when sunlight is more intense.

Melasma gets worse over time with exposure to sunlight. If you are pregnant, particularly in the summer, be sure every single morning to apply a suncreen with an SPF of 15 or greater with zinc, titanium, or Mexoryl and reapply it frequently. You should also wear a hat.

Melasma with oral contraceptives.   This is less of a problem for women forty and over because fewer of us are on oral contraceptives. If you are taking oral contraceptives and begin to develop blotchy brown patches on your face, talk to your dermatologist right away. The sooner the better. The longer you stay on the oral contraceptives, the greater the chance the melasma will become a permanent problem.

Melasma with hormone-replacement therapy.   As we know from the press, hormone-replacement therapy can be a very complicated issue, and I won't go into all the pros and cons and individual and family health risks that need to be considered here. Suffice it to say that, *if* for health reasons you are on hormone replacement therapy, it may be possible to take the HRT in the evening (check with your doctor) instead of the morning, so that the peak levels occur at night. The creams and patches may be slightly more melasma-friendly than the oral versions. The oral versions are cleared in the liver and changed to compounds which may make you more melasma-prone. Take the lowest dose that you can.

If you get melasma from postmenopausal hormone replacement and can't stop the HRT for health reasons, then use sunscreen, stay out of the midday sun, keep your hat on, and talk to your dermatologist about prescription "bleaching" creams. All these simple measures will help to limit the blotchiness of melasma.

Brown Spots due to Acne

Many women, particularly women of color and those with dark hair and dark eyes, develop brown spots on their face after acne or other skin irritations. The medical term for this is *post-inflammatory hyperpigmentation.* The brown spots from acne will fade with time, but it can take months. The postacne brown spots can be there long after the acne has resolved. If you have this kind of spotting after your acne, check for solutions in the treatment section later in this chapter.

Brown Spots due to Picking

I can't tell you how many times I've written in patients' charts "STOP PICKING" in huge capital letters followed by five exclamation points. Now, having said that, have I ever picked something on my face? Of course, everyone has. Picking a little bit every once in a while is absolutely normal. Picking every day so that you are creating scars on your face and brown spots from all the areas that are now healing is *not* normal. You need the care of a dermatologist or psychiatrist if you're picking every day.

REAL-WORLD ADVICE

I'm only forty-two. Why am I getting age spots already? You're getting age spots as a result of the amount of sun damage that you have had and the skin type that you were born with. Even Latino, Asian, or olive Mediterranean skin with enough sun exposure will develop brown spots from sun damage. Sun exposure is cumulative, so it's what you do day after day, year after year that matters. The amount of sun damage you have

---

WAYS TO STOP PICKING

- Put a sticky note on your mirror to remind yourself to stop.
- If you pick at night after you wash your face, try putting concealer over any spots so you won't be bothered by them—the picking is worse than the concealer.
- If you pick unconsciously, ask friends and family to tell you when you're doing it.
- If you pick alone or in the car, put an elastic band on your right wrist to remind you not to.
- If you pick when you're anxious, identify the triggers and reassure yourself instead.
- Get counselling.

---

is also often related to where you grew up. My patients who are from Southern California, for instance, have more sun damage than those who grew up in England.

I have eczema. After the eczema heals, it leaves brown blotches on my face which can sometimes last for months.   The good news is that brown spots resulting from eczema will usually resolve on their own, albeit slowly. You should be treated by your dermatologist with prescription creams for the eczema and the discoloration. If you are sensitive to products, ask your dermatologist for suggestions and avoid any over-the-counter measures other than good moisturizers and sunscreen until you can be seen. Nonprescription "bleaching" creams may irritate your skin further.

TREATING MELASMA AND BROWN SPOTS

If you have melasma from hormones or prior pregnancies, see your dermatologist first. Melasma is the most difficult to treat of these conditions, and you'll need more expert care than you can get with over-the-counter remedies. Also see your dermatologist if you have moderately severe acne or a chronic picking problem. If you have mild blotchiness and brown spots from sun damage or a little acne, however, try over-the-counter products first.

Sunscreen, sunscreen, sunscreen!   You will not have any success treating these if you don't block light. Every time ultraviolet light hits these brown spots it makes them worse. Your sunscreen must block UVA well.

Double sunscreen.   Especially the areas where you have the most blotches. Try using the Colorescience Sunforgetable SPF 30 powder over a cream sunscreen or a mineral pigment sunscreening makeup like Jane Iredale over the sunscreen. Wear a hat to keep the light off those areas if you can.

Nonprescription "bleaching" creams.   These creams don't really "bleach" anything. Instead, they block the production of excess pigment in the skin. The pigment-making cells are like little factories that churn out microscopic brown granules. The bleaching creams partly shut down the factory so less brown pigment granules are made. However, as soon as you stop using the cream, the light can stimulate the cells again and the pigment production may gear up, causing the problem to recur. These work only if your problem is minimal. They all contain 2 percent hydroquinone and have been used for thirty years in various parts of the world.

Prescription "bleaching" creams.   There are a number of different prescription hydroquinone creams, most containing 4 percent hydroquinone (HQ4%) and other active ingredients. The best-known ones are EpiQuin Micro, Tri-Luma Cream, Lustra (in various forms), and Solage. Generic versions are available for less money but have a different base. Your dermatologist can help you select the right one for you.

These creams tend to be expensive and sometimes insurance will not cover them. You might want to clarify with your insurance company ahead of time which creams are covered and which are not. There is also a generic, plain hydroquinone 4 percent, which is inexpensive. However, I and many dermatologists don't prescribe it much because it often causes irritation. If you're using a prescription hydroquinone-based cream and you're getting worse, be sure to stop the cream and call your doctor. The cream shouldn't sting or burn when applied.

The European Union has taken all hydroquinones off their "safe" list, however. Don't use them continuously over large areas or use the hydroquinone products for longer than three to six months without a dermatologist's approval.

Plant-based "bleaching" creams.   There are various plant-based compounds like arbutin, thymol, and kojic acid that inhibit pigment production, too. Generally not as strong as the hydroquinones, they may help if your problem is mild.

REAL-WORLD ADVICE

I have mild acne, but every time I get even one small pimple it leaves a brown spot that seems to last forever. My guess is that you have either dark eyes or dark hair or both. Since it sounds mild, try controlling the acne first with nonprescription products that contain either a little salicylic acid or benzoyl peroxide or both. A good one is Clinique Mild Clarifying Lotion (2 percent salicylic acid). Or try Solvere or Proactiv (available online); they have products with both. These are good for oily skin—they're too drying for other types of skin. Also, one of the over-the-counter bleaching creams with 2 percent hydroquinone could be helpful. Use it for a week or two right after the breakout on the spots only.

My doctor tells me I need to stop picking at my face. Is it true that this is causing brown marks?   Absolutely. Not only does picking at your skin transfer bacteria from your hands to your face, which can result in infections, but picking ruptures the acne down deeper into the skin where it can cause more inflammation. That inflammation can result in more pigment being made, thus the brown spot.

Peels and Microdermabrasion for Melasma and Sun Damage

Both peels and microdermabrasion work by increasing cell turnover, which speeds the transit of that unwanted pigment out of your skin. They can be helpful for all types of brown spots regardless of their origin. Both of them also help to clear up acne if that's part of your underlying problem. Peels in series or deeper peels should be done at a dermatologist's office. For microdermabrasion or peels, go to an experienced (at least five years) aesthetician or nurse.

Microdermabrasion.   Microdermabrasion is a method by which very fine crystals are vacuumed across the skin under pressure with a tiny vacuum-cleaner-like tip. The newer systems don't use crystals but instead, tiny diamond chips embedded in the tip to provide the abrasion. It's nice to use the newer crystal-free system but not essential.

Also, the newer systems offer the ability to infuse therapeutic agents at the same time that the microdermabrasion is being performed. For example, an aesthetician can infuse a solution of salicylic acid, which helps to clean out the pores while the microdermabrasion is working.

Microdermabrasion can cause complications if the microdermabrasion is too aggressive for your skin type.

Depending on how much acne or pigment you have and how sensitive your skin is, approximately five microdermabrasions are done two to four weeks apart, followed by a maintenance treatment about every four to eight weeks.

Light peels.   The best known of these are light glycolic peels. These are usually done either in a salon or more expertly, usually, in a dermatologist's office where the aesthetician is trained to use different strengths of glycolic acid. There are also peels that contain a beta-hydroxy acid like salicylic acid. These peels also take off a few layers of dead skin, help to clean out pores, and are used in a series.

These low-strength gentle acids are stroked onto previously cleansed skin and then left on for several minutes. The acid either self-neutralizes (the one we like in my office is the Vitalize peel) or is neutralized by the nurse or aesthetician performing the treatment. The skin will be slightly pink and feel tight for a few days, and then it will peel, either microscopically or like a mild sunburn.

With light acid peels, however, if the nurse or aesthetician isn't experienced, sometimes the acid can be absorbed more in one spot than another and leave temporary irritation and a dark mark. Darker skin is more susceptible to this than lighter skin. Glycolic peels can also go deep enough that they can occasionally form a blister, but scarring is rare. If you decide to go the peel route, I recommend that you find a dermatologist-supervised nurse or aesthetician experienced in performing these peels.

Trichloroacetic acid (TCA) peels.   Dermatologists have been using TCA peels, a close cousin to vinegar, to do chemical peeling for at least twenty years. Some dermatologists, in fact, still prefer TCA peels to any other modality for treating melasma, usually in combination with prescription creams. TCA peels are excellent and safe in the hands of an experienced dermatologist. This is a good option, particularly if you have severe melasma. The cost generally ranges from three hundred to fifteen hundred dollars, depending on how deep the peel is, the region you live in, and your doctor.

One advantage of a TCA peel is that it can easily be done in your dermatologist's office and doesn't require anesthesiology or any intravenous anesthesia. Deep TCA peels, because of the risk of uneven absorption, blistering, and possible scarring, should be performed only by board-certified dermatologists or plastic surgeons who are experienced in this procedure. There is also a prepeel solution called Jessner's solution, which can be applied before the procedure and allows the TCA to penetrate better. Some physicians will use Jessner's solution as a light peeling agent all by itself.

The other disadvantage is that TCA peels can be mild to moderately uncomfortable. However, with some Tylenol or antiinflammatories, the discomfort is usually minimal and lasts only five to ten minutes.

REAL-WORLD ADVICE

My doctor wants to use liquid nitrogen rather than a peel to get rid of brown spots on my face. What do you think?   For many years, liquid nitrogen was the main treatment available for brown spots. The drawback to this approach is that it often leaves a white area or an uneven blotchy area. For this reason, most dermatologists no longer use liquid nitrogen in this instance. Other treatments provide a better, more even result in the long run.

Lasers for Brown Spots

First of all, if you have melasma, or any darkening that is hormone related, don't allow anyone but an expert to use lasers on your face. Many lasers will make melasma worse, not better, and it is important to go to one of the expert laser centers listed in the back of this book if you're considering laser treatments for melasma.

If you have brown spots as a result of acne or mild picking, lasers may work, but in my opinion they aren't the most cost effective. You can get an excellent result with prescription treatment for your acne, behavior modification for your picking, and a series of light peels or microdermabrasions for the brown spots. The exception might be if you have brown spots due to both sun damage and the acne pigmentation problem. Then using the laser to take care of both might be a good idea.

So, which laser should you use for brown spots due to sun damage? This question really depends on which skin type you are. Types 1 and 2 are types that are pale and burn easily in the sun. Types 3 and 4 are skin types that are much less likely to burn (but still can occasionally) and usually have some olive, dark gold, mocha tones in them. Types 5 and 6 are darker, more cocoa to chocolate shades, and almost never burn and are not very prone to this type of sun damage.

Lasers for skin types 1 and 2.   There are a number of lasers that work well for brown spots due to sun damage. I still prefer photorejuvenation, which is done with an Intense Pulsed Light device (IPL), a laser cousin, particularly for younger patients. I prefer these lasers for sun-damaged skin because they take care of brown spots, any red, blotchy areas or dilated blood vessels, and improve texture and in addition build collagen. Most people with sun-damaged skin have all three of these problems and can benefit from this type of treatment. Fractional lasers like the Fraxel may be a better choice if you have wrinkles or acne scarring in addition to brown spots. IPLs and other lasers can make melasma worse, so consult only expert cosmetic dermatologists for that problem. Lasers like a Q-switched YAG, remove only the brown spots without providing the other benefits.

How is the laser treatment done?   The doctor or nurse passes the handset over the skin being treated and the light from the IPL/laser hits the brown spots (or dilated blood vessels) and damages them. The age spot or sun spot looks slightly darker for about a week and then begins to lighten and then gradually sheds or peels off. These laser treatments are done in a series, usually approximately three to five times about a month apart and then once or twice a year for maintenance depending on your sun exposure.

Lasers for skin types 3 and 4.   Darker skin types are harder to treat correctly. The key is the laser system being used but also the expertise of the laser clinic doctors and nurses who are treating you. See chapter 16 on how to find a good laser center and a good doctor.

Lasers for skin types 5 and 6.   Darker skin types may need different lasers to prevent laser burns. Go to a center that is experienced with darker skin types, since the last thing you would want is to get a burn or to have your brown spots get worse. See chapter 16 for more information.

THE BOTTOM LINE ON BLOTCHINESS, BROWN SPOTS, AND AGE SPOTS

- Be sure to talk to your doctor about any suspicious spot on your face. Malignant melanoma, which is a deadly and possibly fatal type of skin cancer, can occur on the face and can begin in something that even looks like a freckle. So, if you see any skin changes, moles, freckles, or growths that you're not sure about, be sure to see a dermatologist for a skin cancer check prior to undertaking any cosmetic treatments.
- Use a good sunscreen every morning that blocks Ultraviolet-A (UVA) and UVB radiation. These are sunscreens containing zinc, titanium, or Mexoryl.
- If your problem is minimal and of short duration, you can try over-the-counter "bleaching" creams. Remember these don't really bleach anything, they just turn off the pigment-making cells temporarily. Most of these contain 2 percent hydroquinone.
- If you have melasma or moderate or severe problems with brown spots, then consult your dermatologist; you'll need expert advice on prescription bleaching creams, peels or microdermabrasion, and possibly laser treatment for your problem.
- Using lasers to treat brown spots, especially in darker skin types, should be done only in dermatologists' offices where experts are

experienced treating darker skin. Particularly with melasma, lasers can make the problem worse.

REDNESS AND DILATED BLOOD VESSELS

Another common concern among women is the redness and dilated blood vessels that often appear on the other side of forty. Here are some of their frequent comments and questions:

- "Do you think the three triple vente lattes that I drink a day could be aggravating my rosacea?"
- "Are there any foods that will help these broken blood vessels on my face?"
- "What products should I use if I have rosacea?"
- "How can I get rid of this redness?"

Redness and Enlarged Blood Vessels on the Face

Flushing.   Just because you flush and blush doesn't always mean you have rosacea. Many of us flush and blush with exercise, heat, or stressful situations. The difference with rosacea is that you might start to flush more and more frequently and with certain triggers. Then, the flushing lasts longer and pretty soon becomes kind of a permanent flush. Acne-like pimples may develop. These signs may mean that you are developing rosacea.

Almost everyone who gets rosacea has a history of flushing and blushing, but not everyone who flushes and blushes gets rosacea. If you're not sure if your flushing is rosacea related, make an appointment with your dermatologist to discuss it.

Rosacea.   Rosacea is a condition that begins as a tendency to flush and blush and progresses to persistent redness and slight swelling across the bridge of the nose, cheeks, forehead or chin. As rosacea progresses, pimples may appear, pores enlarge and become bumpy (sebaceous hy-

CAUSES OF FLUSHING

- rosacea
- stress/anxiety
- menopausal hormones
- exercise
- alcohol
- sun damage
- allergies
- rare endocrine diseases

perplasia), and small, dilated blood vessels appear. These blood vessels, particularly around the nose, can become quite large over time.

Unlike acne, there are no blackheads. In very advanced cases, a condition called rhinophyma (the W. C. Fields nose) may develop. This occurs when the oil glands and the blood vessels on the nose enlarge so much that it becomes very bulbous and red.

Initially, the redness and acne-like breakouts of rosacea may come and go. You may not even realize you need treatment. Keep in mind that about half the rosacea sufferers have eye symptoms too—many may experience some burning and grittiness of the eye (called conjunctivitis) or inflammation or swelling of the eyelid area. See your ophthalmologist if that's the case.

Rosacea gradually becomes worse without treatment, and after a while becomes more permanent. So, if your skin does not return to its original color or you start to see pimples or enlarged blood vessels, definitely see your dermatologist. The key to successful management of rosacea is early diagnosis and treatment. Your dermatologist will discuss lifestyle and dietary interventions as well as prescription treatments for rosacea.

POSSIBLE DIETARY CAUSES OF ROSACEA

Depending on the list you look at, there may be twenty-five or thirty different foods and drinks associated with rosacea. The question is, do you experience an increase in your symptoms when you eat or drink one of these? If you don't, don't worry about it. Here are the most common:

- alcohol
- coffee
- tea, depending on type
- hot liquids, in general
- soy
- nuts
- tomatoes
- citrus fruits

Redness and large blood vessels due to sun damage.　We've talked a lot about sun damage. But one of the things it can do, in addition to causing brown spots, is to enlarge the small blood vessels of the face. This causes a red and veiny appearance on the face. Some people with sun damage never develop this problem—they just get brown and blotchy. This red type of sun damage occurs on the neck—hence, the term *redneck.* It can also occur on the chest.

Other causes of redness.　There are other problems that can cause redness on the face and flushing. These include systemic lupus and other autoimmune disorders, menopause, some thyroid problems, special sun-sensitivity problems, and some gland (endocrine) disorders. These are why it's important to see a dermatologist for correct diagnosis. If you suspect one of these, also make an appointment with your primary care doctor for a thorough exam and labs.

Lasers to Treat Redness and Dilated Blood Vessels

Before you have any laser treatment for redness, see a dermatologist to understand the cause of your redness. You don't want to spend money on a series of laser treatments for redness, only to find your redness reappearing months later due to untreated rosacea.

Lasers for redness and broken blood vessels on the face have evolved remarkably over the last ten years, and redness can be dramatically reduced by lasers with little downtime. Most patients come into the office, have a treatment, put on makeup, and walk back out to their normal activities.

The best lasers for this problem are pulsed dye lasers (in the 595 nanometer range) or the intense pulse light devices (IPLs) that we've talked about before for photorejuvenation. They both work well and have different advantages and disadvantages depending on what other problems you might have.

If you have sun damage and brown spots in addition to being red, then the IPL may be better. It will take care of both problems at the same time. I use an IPL most frequently because most of my patients have both rosacea and sun damage.

If you are younger and/or have only redness and veins and not much sun damage, the pulsed dye laser may be a better choice. Again, the training, judgment, experience, and ethics of the doctor supervising or using the laser are more important than exactly what model of laser is used.

REAL-WORLD ADVICE

Can I go back to work right after my laser treatment?   Generally, yes. After treatments you may look like you have a light sunburn for a few hours or a day or two. Sometimes there's mild swelling for several days. The redness that is being treated may look a little blotchier than usual, but foundation or concealer usually covers it nicely. Many doctors will limit exercise for a few days or a week after a treatment. Since there can be some mild swelling and redness, you might want to schedule your first

WHEN TO RUN OUT THE DOOR!

- If anyone tries to use a laser on your face or around your eyes without eye shields placed over your eye
- If a laser is being done directly on your eyelid and a contact-lens-style eye shield is not in place
- If they can't answer your questions about eye protection— certain lasers done around the eye can cause blindness

treatment at the end of a day before a quiet evening. Then, once you know how you respond, you'll be more confident about what you can do immediately after a treatment. Most of my patients (and myself), just put on a little makeup and go right back to activities and work.

Do the treatments hurt?   Most patients tolerate treatments easily. The laser feels like a mild rubber band snapped against the skin. There's also a bright flash of light with the IPL devices—your eyes will be covered, but some patients are surprised at the flash.

How many treatments will I need?   Usually getting rid of most of the redness or dilated blood vessels will take three to six treatments. This is the repair phase. If you have just a few small vessels, one to three treatments might be enough. If you're extremely red and have been so for many years, five to eight treatments might be needed. Ask your dermatologist for a rough estimate of how many you might need. Remember, though, if you engage in a lot of habits that induce flushing (including good habits, such as exercising) you may need a few extra treatments or more maintenance.

Are the results permanent?   No. Nothing in the universe, including the effect of any cosmetic treatment, is permanent. The most common scenario is to need one or two maintenance treatments a year depending on how much you flush and blush as well as alcohol use, menopause, exercise, and other individual variables.

How much do laser treatments for redness cost?   Costs vary according to the area being treated, where you live and the skill of and the demand for your particular dermatologist. A general ballpark figure for treating your whole face is three hundred to eight hundred dollars per treatment or fifteen hundred to four thousand dollars for a series of five. Spas will often offer inexpensive treatments but the lasers they use are weaker versions (in most states) and their "technicians" often have no medical training other than a one- or two-day laser course.

I'm getting pretty red. When should I consider getting laser treatments?   When your flushing is bad enough that it's interfering with your work or social life (for example, if you're avoiding speaking in public because you're afraid you might flush or blush), then consider getting a series of laser treatments. Also, if you feel you have to pile on the makeup in the morning just to feel presentable, it's time to consider spending the money on laser treatments.

I'm a little afraid of laser treatments. Are they really safe?   They are very safe if you go to a reputable laser center run by a dermatologist who has experience with lasers. It is fine for an RN, ARNP or PA-C closely supervised by a doctor to do laser treatments as well. I strongly believe, though, that lasers should be used only by medical personnel, meaning doctors, PAs, ARNPs, or nurses. Many medi-spas hire staff without medical training including aestheticians, train them for a day or two, and then turn them loose on the public with a laser. They often have very little on-site supervision, or the supervising doctor is not even a dermatologist. Complications with lasers can occur. I know because I have seen them year after year in my office. We often get people referred who are burned or otherwise disfigured by laser treatments done by people who are either poorly trained or poorly supervised. Beware of the term *laser technician*. This usually means that the person using the laser on you has no medical training.

I'm afraid I'll spend a lot of money getting my redness and veins treated and then not get much effect. I'm on a budget and laser treatments are expensive for me.   Again, this is where you want to look for a well-established reputable laser center. While no center will absolutely guarantee results, a good laser center with long-term roots in the community will want to make sure that you are happy with your laser treatments. They will not allow you to spend a lot of money and go away without a great (not perfect) result. Look for a practice that has roots in the community and a good reputation.

THE BOTTOM LINE ON REDNESS

- Make all the right lifestyle changes you can reasonably make and try to be consistent. You'll save yourself time and money in the long run.
- If you suspect you have rosacea, be sure to see a dermatologist, since controlling this skin disease is usually not complicated.
- If you have medications from your doctor for rosacea, use them! If you have rosacea, you'll usually have it for twenty to thirty years. So don't go off the medication just because you are doing well. Using the medications will help prevent the progression of the disease even if it doesn't immediately make you look less red.
- Use your sunscreen every day to avoid aggravating the redness and blood vessels with sun damage.
- After you've controlled your rosacea, a series of three to six laser treatments followed by one or two maintenance treatments a year will give you good results and is worth the money and time.

10

UNWANTED HAIR, BUMPS, MOLES, AND SCARS ON THE FACE

The most common error made in matters of appearance is the belief that one should disdain the superficial and let the true beauty of one's soul shine through. If there are places on your body where this is a possibility, you are not attractive—you are leaking.

—Fran Lebowitz

No one wants her face to look like a topographical map. When we're young, our pores are small, and moles or growths are minimal. As time goes on, pore size increases, oil glands enlarge, and those moles that used to be small become more protuberant. And, if there is any acne scarring, valleys and pits may disrupt the smooth surface of our skin.

That smoothness of skin, its texture, is what gives it its glow. The medical way to describe glowing skin is to say that it has high reflectivity—the smoother our skin is, the more reflectivity there will be. As we accumulate those lumps and bumps over time and the dead skin layer on top thickens, the reflectivity of our skin decreases. This decline in reflectivity is one thing that makes older skin look, well, older. Restoring the smoothness of your skin can help restore that youthful glow of reflectivity.

Here's what women often say:

- "These moles that I've had for years seem like they are getting larger. Can they be removed without a scar?"
- "I can't stand these chin (or upper-lip) hairs anymore."

- "What are all these little bumps all over my forehead and cheeks?"
- "I have acne scars."
- "My pores are getting bigger, and my skin is still oily even though I'm fifty."
- "I have this spot that won't heal."

Whether you have old acne scars or just a few moles that stick out, there has never been a better time to get your skin smoother again. There are many more options available now than there were even five years ago. Thankfully, the goal of smooth, even-textured skin is attainable with some time, effort, and money.

UNWANTED HAIR ON THE FACE

Problem: Too much hair on the face

Best Solutions: Laser hair removal, electrolysis, Vaniqa cream

Laser Hair Removal

Laser hair removal has become very effective in the past ten years. Often the preferred method of hair removal now, it's safe, effective, and more permanent than any other method such as waxing, plucking, shaving, and electrolysis. The easiest person to treat for laser hair removal has darker hair on lighter skin. But there are now lasers that do a good job with dark hair on dark skin.

How does it work? The laser emits a very specific beam of light at a wavelength that is targeted at melanin. Melanin is the material that gives color to our hair and skin. The laser beam passes through the skin and is absorbed by the melanin in the hair follicle. Therefore, the ideal candidate for this procedure has hair that is darker than her skin color. If the skin and hair color are too similar, it confuses some lasers. Darker skin needs "long-wave" hair-removal lasers like the YAG laser. They are safer if you have darker skin because they won't "burn" the skin trying to get rid of the hair.

WHEN IS LASER HAIR REMOVAL MORE DIFFICULT?

- if you have hormonal abnormalities like irregular periods or polycystic ovaries
- if your hair is blond or white
- if it's hard for you to make time for the initial series of five or six monthly appointments
- if your hair isn't darker than your skin color
- if you can't get yourself to stop tanning

Does it hurt? There may be mild discomfort during the treatment, but most patients tolerate laser hair removal very easily. Treatments can take from minutes to an hour or more, depending on the size of the treatment area. Your doctor may also use a topical numbing treatment or a cooling machine that blows very cold air to make the laser treatment more comfortable.

How many treatments will I need? After three to seven treatments initially, most women report that their expectations have been met and the hair growth pattern is much, much less. In some areas, in addition to the decrease in the number of hairs, the hairs become very fine and light in color. No laser clinic should claim that all of the hairs will be permanently eradicated. Most patients will need a touch-up several times a year to maintain the improvement.

Expect to need more treatments if you have any history of irregular periods, polycystic ovary disease, gray or white hairs or a family history of excessive hair. About 5 percent of patients are resistant to any type of hair removal laser. It is very important to have a realistic expectation regarding individual results of hair removal. *No hair-removal system anywhere is "permanent."*

Electrolysis

This is a method by which a tiny electric needle is manually pushed down into the hair follicle to injure the follicle. It works but is best for women with just a few hairs or for gray or very blond hair. It can be painful, time consuming, and if done badly, leave permanent scars. Best are operators who have been in business at least five years and who come from a medical background. Look for an RN or MA degree.

Vaniqa Cream

This is a prescription cream that slows and inhibits hair growth on the face. It's best for women who have fuzzy, blond hairs that are becoming too thick or noticeable. Apply it twice a day. It takes four to six months to see results.

LUMPS AND BUMPS ON THE FACE

There are different types of lumps and bumps, and I'll briefly mention several here. Keep in mind that self-diagnosis, however, is never a good idea. If you're not sure what something is, be sure to have your dermatologist check it. Skin cancers can look fine to an untrained eye. It's important to be absolutely sure that that bump on your face isn't a skin cancer.

Milia

Milia is a type of very small cyst which hardens in a pore under the skin. Most of us have had at least one of these. They look like they are maybe a whitehead or small pimple. But when we try to squeeze them (since we're human), they don't come out.

Milia can be difficult to get rid of on your own. Squeezing them can cause so much trauma that your skin actually looks worse. Your dermatologist or an experienced aesthetician can remove these milia easily with a special tool. Make an appointment to get them taken care of professionally rather than traumatize yourself.

TYPES OF BENIGN AND HARMLESS FACIAL BUMPS OR LESIONS

- sebaceous hyperplasia—overgrown oil glands
- moles—the medical term is *nevi*
- milia—a hard, deep plug in a pore
- seborrheic keratoses—coin-sized, flat tan or brown spots
- fibrous papules—small, firm bumps usually on the nose

Treatment. Your dermatologist will make a tiny, almost invisible, puncture over the top of the milia and then use a tool called a comedone extractor to pop the milia out. Afterward there may be a little bit of crusting or blood around the area for a day or two so don't plan this immediately before an important function or presentation. Also, creams in the vitamin-A family, such as Renova, Retin-A, or tretinoin, if used for a month or so before the extraction, help to loosen the milia and make them easier to remove.

Enlarged Oil Glands (Sebaceous Hyperplasia)

These show up as small, soft, yellowish or off-white bumps on the skin. The most common areas for them are between the eyebrows, the forehead, the nose, sometimes around the mouth, and occasionally around the cheeks if your cheeks are oily. Unlike milia, sebaceous hyperplasia (SH) aren't hard. They tend to be the same texture as the skin. Also, if you look very closely you may see a small pore in the center of the bump—they're basically just oil glands that have enlarged over time.

Many of us have one or two of these little bumps on the forehead or around the nose where most of our oil glands are concentrated. However, if you have very oily skin along with large pores (and often acne problems), you may have a lot of these bumps. As you accumulate these over the years, they will give your face a bumpy appearance.

Treatment. There are a number of treatment options for SH, but I prefer to use electrocautery with a little surgical curette. The electrocautery looks like a small electric pencil and essentially melts and flattens the enlarged oil gland. Then a tiny, sharp loop smoothes the skin even more. The goal is to flatten and smooth the SH, not to cut it out (that would leave scarring). It does leave a small crust while it's healing, which takes about three to seven days depending on the size of the spot. Usually the procedure can be done with no scarring at all. SHs will slowly regrow over a period of years, and maintenance is needed.

Other treatment options include resurfacing lasers, but there is more recovery time with those. But if you have acne scarring in addition to a lot of SH, this may be a good option for you. The fractional resurfacing lasers may be useful for this problem, but we just don't have enough research data yet. These are expensive lasers so unless money is no object, I would recommend waiting for another year or two for more information. I do not recommend liquid nitrogen for the bumps of sebaceous hyperplasia—it causes too much irritation and can cause white spots.

Barnacles (Seborrheic Keratoses)

These look like small to medium brownish, dry growths or rough patches on the face (and body). They're usually raised from the skin a little bit and can look almost "stuck on." Sometimes the surface appears warty and waxy, but these are not warts! They often grow slowly but can become quite large over many years. The color, although usually brown, can range from flesh color to a very dark brown, almost black, particularly if you have dark eyes or dark hair.

They're called barnacles or SKs, partly because they look stuck on to you like a barnacle and partly because it's just too cumbersome to say "seborrheic keratoses" every time we see one of these common benign growths. Be sure to have your dermatologist look at these before they are removed. Don't assume that a growth isn't cancerous on your own.

Almost everyone over the age of forty has at least a few of these some-where on their face or body. They can occur anywhere, including the face, scalp, trunk, arms, or legs. There is no evidence, by the way, that barnacles found in the scalp are caused by hair coloring.

Keep in mind that while the evaluation of these is covered by your in-surance (to make sure it's not skin cancer), the removal of these is cos-metic. They are benign and not any threat to your health, which is why most insurance plans, including Medicare, won't pay for their removal. The cost for removing these varies from office to office, but most offices charge a very reasonable fee to have them removed (we charge anywhere from $25 to $125 depending on how many there are).

Treatment. The most common method for removing these is to spray liquid nitrogen on them. Liquid nitrogen comes in air-tight insulated cans and is either sprayed on with a tiny nozzle or applied with a cotton-tipped applicator for a variable amount of time depending on the thickness of the growth. Even though it's very cold, liquid nitrogen can give a burning sensa-tion on application that can be uncomfortable for a few hours or even a day or two. You can take Tylenol or ibuprofen if that's the case.

After the treatment, the site will usually get red and irritated around the base, almost like an insect bite. Then it will crust over or even occa-sionally blister a little. It usually takes one to two weeks for the sites to heal. Occasionally there may be a temporary pink or brown mark at the site for a month or two after removal. It will go away.

The other option for removal is the electrocautery and curette method mentioned above to treat enlarged oil glands. I prefer to use this method on the face (as opposed to liquid nitrogen) because it heals faster and there is less risk of uneven pigment or scarring. You might ask your dermatologist which method she prefers.

Small Bumps (Fibrous Papules) on the Nose

There are many different growths that can occur on the nose, including skin cancers, sebaceous hyperplasia (enlarged oil glands), moles, and also fibrous papules. Fibrous papules (FPs) show up usually as reddish or flesh colored, firm, small bumps about a quarter of an inch in diameter. Even though these are common and benign, it's very important to have your dermatologist check them. Certain skin cancers can look very similar to these. If there is any question that the bump might be a skin cancer, it will be biopsied. This is fine since it removes the lesion and also allows the pathologist to examine the tissue. Again, your dermatologist can advise you.

BENIGN MOLES ON THE FACE

Problem: Raised or flat moles on the face that are a cosmetic issue
Best Solution: Surgical excision by a dermatologist

Many of my patients want to know if it's possible to remove large moles on the face without leaving a big scar. The answer is yes; it's often quite easy to surgically remove moles, especially raised ones, without leaving a noticeable scar. You'll always be trading the mole for a scar, but the question is, is it a good trade? If the scar is barely visible, and the mole is quite raised and noticeable, then you'll probably think it's a good trade. If a mole is tiny, it may not be such a benefit to have it removed.

There are several different kinds of moles, each of which may call for a different kind of removal and have its own healing process. The best thing to do is to see a dermatologist for an examination of your particular moles. Most of the time you don't need a plastic surgeon to remove a mole on the face, unless it's in a particularly bad spot or especially large.

Keep in mind that insurance companies tend to view cosmetic mole removal as medically unnecessary. Most won't cover it. Dermatologists charge a fee for mole removal, anywhere from $250 to $800 for each mole. Plastic surgeons will be generally more expensive. A pathology slide will be made and read after the excision to make sure that the mole is not precancerous or cancerous.

REAL-WORLD ADVICE

I have a large mole on the bridge of my nose. Can this be easily removed?   Surprisingly, the nose is one of the easier places on the face to achieve a good result when doing a shave excision. It often heals flat and almost invisibly. If you are young, it may grow back, and you may need to have it removed again.

I have a lot—and I mean a lot—of enlarged oil glands on my face. Should I get them removed?   Without seeing you, it's a little tough. But I would say yes, with the understanding that there will be some healing time and that you may need two or three sessions to remove them all. I usually treat my patients in the winter (no sun for a month) and on a Thursday. That way they can take Friday and possibly Monday off work and be back by Tuesday with makeup (not looking perfect but okay). If you are in television, you may need one to two weeks to be "camera ready."

PORE SIZE

Problem: Enlarged pores
Best Solution: Nothing is great, but some lasers may be helpful

Pore size is decided by a combination of the skin type that you inherited from your family, the amount of oil your skin produces, and whether or not you have acne or other skin diseases. Almost everyone is oilier and has larger pores through the forehead, nose, and chin area (the T zone). Children have tiny, almost invisible pores because their skin has not yet begun to produce oil.

Notwithstanding what you may read on the Internet, I'm sorry to say that there is no reliable and effective way to shrink large pores—yet. The Fraxel laser may be helpful, but there isn't enough data yet on it. This is an exciting area, and I'm hoping that in the next few years there will be more effective laser treatments for large pores and excessive oil. Photorejuvenation with an IPL or long-wave lasers like the Aramis may shrink pores slightly because they decrease oil production. This is a temporary effect.

In the absence of tried-and-true laser systems, you can always cover your pores with makeup. I think the best ones for oily skin and large pores are the powder-based mineral makeups, like the Jane Iredale line or Bare Escentuals. They give good coverage and decrease the visibility of the pores without adding oil to the skin. In fact, the powders are a bit drying, which is good. Also, microdermabrasion and light peels help to keep the pores clean and dead skin from building up, both of which may help to keep pores looking smaller.

FIXING ACNE SCARRING

Problem: Acne scars not treated in younger years are looking worse
Best Solutions: Subscision or lasers

Acne scars tend to look worse as we age because the skin supporting the scars becomes less elastic and firm. This allows the scar to sag more. To understand what might work best for your type of scarring, you need to look at your face and decide what types of scars you have. The most common type of acne scars are those shallow rolling scars, which are also the easiest to treat. Often, your dermatologist may combine different types of treatment to get the best results possible.

Fractional Laser Resurfacing

This is a relatively new type of laser treatment in the battle against acne scars. Some centers have posted very nice results with this type of laser. It does, however, happen to be expensive. If you need your whole face done, it will run between one thousand and two thousand dollars per treatment. Since you'll need three to five treatments, that can get you up toward three thousand to eight thousand dollars. Acne-scar subscision is usually less expensive. Sometimes combining the two is best. You could have one or two sessions of subscision followed by one or two fractional laser resurfacings, or vice versa.

Acne Scar Subscision

Subscision is best for the rolling type of scar. Your doctor will numb the area first and then push a special type of needle through the skin down to the area where the scar tissue is and then work the special needle around

HERE ARE DIFFERENT TYPES OF ACNE SCARRING:

- Ice-pick scars. These are the narrow but deep scars that sometimes look like a very large pore but go deep into the skin.
- Boxcar scars. These look like someone poked a tiny box into the skin because the walls of the scar are vertical.
- Rolling scars. These are shallow scars with a broad base.

underneath the scar to break up the abnormal collagen layer. As the area heals, the new collagen formation during the healing process will push the base of the scar up.

There is a lot of bruising after each treatment, so plan on at least a week off after the subscision. Usually a series of one to three treatments will produce the best results. These can be alternated with laser treatments to optimize results even more. A subscision treatment could cost anywhere from $250 to $1,500 per treatment depending on how many scars there are.

Traditional Laser Resurfacing

The carbon dioxide (CO_2) lasers and the erbium YAG (Er:YAG) are the two main lasers used for resurfacing. With both these lasers, tiny micron-width layers of skin are removed until the laser surgeon reaches a level that will have the best effect on the scar without risking complications. This is both a science and an art and takes considerable experience. Results are usually excellent.

The problem with this type of laser is there is a risk of infection, a risk of scarring, and a risk of the skin growing back with a lighter or darker color temporarily or permanently after the resurfacing. Also, the recovery time for this is long. Plan on at least two weeks off work, and even then your skin may be red to pink for many months after that. Also, the pool of laser surgeons who do enough of this procedure to be really good at it is shrinking. Make sure you go to a nationally recognized laser center (see chapter 17) for this type of procedure.

Punch Grafting

Punch grafting is best for icepick-type scars that are narrow but deep. First the scar is excised completely with a tiny circular tool just slightly larger than the scar. Then, either the small hole is closed with sutures and allowed to heal, or a tiny piece of skin is taken from behind the ear or another site and put into the hole where the acne scar once was. After the area has healed, some fractional or traditional resurfacing can be done to blend the color of the skin throughout the area that was punch grafted. Laser resurfacing works well if the acne scars aren't too deep.

Filler Injections

Fillers work by being injected into the scar to raise the depressed area up to the surface of the skin. The hyaluronic-acid fillers like Restylane or Juvederm may be helpful, but they can flow around the scar instead of into it. I prefer to use CosmoPlast, which is a more modern version of collagen. It flows nicely into scars. The main disadvantage of fillers is that they're temporary. You would need to have the injections repeated every four to nine months.

REAL-WORLD ADVICE

Is acne scarring preventable now?   This question is for your children. Yes, for the most part it is. Since the type of acne that causes scars is usually cystic or pustular acne, if it is caught early and treated aggressively, scarring can by and large be prevented. With cystic acne, in particular, a course of Accutane is still the most effective treatment. A combination of oral antibiotics or oral contraceptives, acne laser treatments, and an acne prescription cream or gel can also stop the acne in its tracks before it starts to cause scarring. Take your children to a dermatologist if they have anything more than mild acne.

WHEN TO BE CONCERNED ABOUT SKIN CANCER

Skin cancers can be more difficult to diagnose than you might think. They are great mimickers, and some skin cancers can look completely innocent. They can also grow so slowly that you think that they can't possibly be a skin cancer.

The take-home message is that any skin growth that is new, bleeding, itching, growing, easily traumatized, looks like an enlarging mole or an enlarging freckle, or even just shows up as a slightly scaly spot that just doesn't go away after a couple of months—all of these should be checked by your dermatologist.

Most primary care doctors are not particularly good at diagnosing skin cancers, especially in the early stages. The vast majority of primary care doctors (internists and family practice doctors), receive almost no training in dermatology. These doctors will recognize a skin cancer once it's more advanced, but why wait? See a dermatologist because you will get a more accurate diagnosis.

Most skin cancers on the face can be treated very effectively if caught early. Scars can usually be kept to a minimum. Early diagnosis is important. Even the most deadly of skin cancers, malignant melanoma, is very curable with a surgery if caught early. If you do have a skin cancer, you may be referred to a special skin-cancer surgeon called a Mohs surgeon. This type of surgery was named after dermatologist Dr. Frederick Mohs.

THE BOTTOM LINE

- See your dermatologist about any suspicious growth on your face.
- Most unwanted hair on the face can be easily removed with lasers.

- Most raised moles on the face can be removed now with minimal scarring, so don't hesitate to talk to your dermatologist about them if they're troubling you.
- There is still no perfect treatment to decrease pore size, but several newer laser systems that help to shrink oil glands and decrease oil are looking promising.
- There are many different ways to treat acne scarring now. Your dermatologist can tell you about those and about how to combine several methods for the best result.
- Many small benign growths on the face can be easily treated by your dermatologist.

PART FOUR
FOCUS ON TIME
AND MONEY

11

HELP ME!
I HAVE A BIG EVENT!

As any jazz musician knows, it takes flexibility and adaptability
for improvisation to create beauty.
—Doc Childre

This chapter focuses on time—getting ready for the big milestone events in your life within a few weeks, a month, a year. The next chapter, chapter 12, focuses on money—how to achieve your goals whether you have a tight budget or unlimited cash!

What sort of milestone events or major life changes are you thinking about? Some women have an important birthday, like the big five-oh or the big six-oh, approaching. Maybe you have a second wedding or a honeymoon on the horizon. Or perhaps you're preparing for a college or high school reunion or a daughter's wedding. Did you just get promoted or make a career change? Or, like many women, have you simply resolved that it's time to get a new look for a "new you"?

I'm going to make some assumptions that underlie the recommendations in this chapter. First, I'm going to assume you're highly motivated to improve the health and beauty of your skin prior to this event. Second, I'm going to assume that money is not tight but is also not flowing out of your pockets. And third, I'm going to assume that you're starting almost from ground zero.

Remember, your skin is an organ like your heart, your largest organ, in fact. You wouldn't expect to have a healthy heart without some good basic health habits. Good health habits go a long way toward having beautiful, healthy skin, too. See chapter 13 for more detailed information on food and lifestyle, but suffice it to say that daily exercise and foods rich in whole grains, vegetables, fruits, high-quality protein and small amounts of healthy fats will help to make your skin *glow*. And don't forget hair and makeup, which may become necessary to complement your healthier, younger-looking skin!

I HAVE ONE MONTH—YIKES!

So you need to get busy—right away. This will be a pretty intense month, but you can make a significant difference in your skin if you follow this plan or an individualized version of it depending on what you and your doctor decide.

Let's pretend that your old college roommate just called to invite you and two other friends to spend a week in Paris in an apartment she has rented. You want to look great and have a wonderful time!

Let's take a minute first to talk about what you *can't* do in a month. Realistically, you can't do a series of laser treatments. You just won't see significant enough results in a month to make it worth starting the series. You also don't want to tackle any treatments that need to develop over time, like Sculptra or even Thermage. Even though with Thermage you might see a little bit of tightening initially, you won't see the full results for four to six months. You need treatments that will give you a lot of short-term bang for your buck.

Assume you'll need approximately two appointments per week for this one-month period with a time commitment of approximately two to four hours per week. Costs will usually run between one thousand to three thousand dollars for the above, depending on your age and how much you need to do.

IN ONE MONTH YOU CAN . . . (FOR EXAMPLE)

- improve your surface texture and your "glow" factor with new products
- improve your texture and "glow" with a light peel or micro-dermabrasion
- relax frown lines, crow's feet, and neck lines with Botox
- fill in the lines from your nose to your mouth and your mouth to your chin
- fill upper-lip lines and improve lip contour and volume
- clean out pores and improve acne

Week 1 Goals *(The Busiest Week)*

- find a great cosmetic dermatologist and make an appointment
- find a good aesthetician and make appointments
- buy your new products
- get a microdermabrasion or light peel at the end of this week
- start walking twenty to thirty minutes a day
- eat whole grains, veggies, fresh fruit, olive oil, fish, and lean meat, and a small amount of dark (70 percent or greater) chocolate (for fun)—think lots of color

Finding a great dermatologist fast (you have only one month!). This is a little tough because many good dermatologists are booked months in advance. Call all your friends, including any doctors with whom you have a good relationship, and ask them to recommend the best cosmetic dermatologists in town: call the dermatologist right away! If he or she is fully booked, what do you do? You have only one month. Here are some tips that may help:

- Explain why you need the appointment. Most people who work in medical offices really do want to help you if they can.
- Try calling the dermatologist's office every morning about 9:30 or 10:00 a.m. Most of the cancellations for the day come in by then.
- Ask if you can be put on a cancellation list.
- Be flexible with your time if you're asking to get in right away.
- Always be nice. Yelling, threatening, name dropping (to excess), and other unpleasant behaviors won't help!

What to say to the dermatologist's schedulers. When you make your dermatology appointment, give them a sense right away for the extent of the treatment you're looking for. Tell them, for instance, that you'd like to treat your frown lines and the crow's feet around your eyes (Botox) and that you'd like to fill the lines from your nose to mouth (nasolabial fold) and mouth to chin (marionette's lines) with Juvederm or Restylane. And if you want your lips fuller or your upper lips lines treated, be sure to mention that too. Expect to spend one thousand to twenty-five hundred dollars for the Botox and the filler.

Remember: no aspirin, Advil/ibuprofen, or Aleve/naprosyn one-week prior to any injection because they'll cause bruising (Tylenol is okay). Don't treat any horizontal forehead lines unless the dermatologist is an expert. The last thing you want is to have your eyebrows drooping or your forehead feeling heavy right before a big event.

Finding a good aesthetician fast. Your dermatologist's office may have an aesthetician who works with her or him, in which case they're probably well-skilled and a good bet for the aesthetician part of this program. If not, ask your dermatologist for a recommendation or ask your friends with great skin whom they work with. You may need to apply some of the same strategies mentioned above to get in to see a great aesthetician on short notice. They can get very booked as well.

Next, set up weekly appointments with your aesthetician for weeks one, two, three, and four. For the aesthetician appointments, schedule a gentle microdermabrasion or a light peel in weeks one and three with hydrating facials in weeks two and four. The microdermabrasion (or light peels) will clean out your pores, exfoliate well, and get your circulation going and your cells more active (the "glow"). The facials will help keep you well hydrated because the microdermabrasions can be somewhat drying. Your aesthetician can adjust these suggestions to your skin type.

By the end of week one, you should have your dermatology appointment set up and your first appointment with your aesthetician at the end of the week.

Update your skin-care regimen. If you already are using good products, stay with them! If you're not, then consider these simple changes to start out. Consistency is the key. Don't change your new regimen unless your skin gets irritated.

These products, many mentioned in chapter 1, are available in the drugstore or online. If your appointment with your dermatologist falls in the first part of week two, you could choose to wait for recommendations from him/her. But if you want to get started sooner—remember you have only one month!—here's what you could buy:

- Use a gentle cleanser—Dove for Sensitive Skin, Cetaphil Liquid Cleanser, or Éminence Lemon Cleanser (organic – available online) are all fine. Wash your face morning and night.
- Use a good moisturizer—Oil of Olay (drugstore), Cetaphil (drugstore), SkinCeuticals Emollience (online). Any moisturizer that doesn't clog your pores is okay.
- Under your moisturizer or sunscreen in the morning, use a good-quality antioxidant—SkinCeuticals C E Ferulic or Cellex-C (online). Replenix with polyphenols is another good antioxidant.
- Apply a UVA/UVB blocking sunscreen, preferably one with zinc, over the vitamin-C serum and your moisturizer every morning. If you have slightly oily skin, eliminate the moisturizer step and just use the sunscreen. Most good-quality sunscreens have a moisturizing base.
- At night, cleanse and moisturize as above.

- Use your Renova (prescription only) or SkinMedica Retinol Complex (online) at night.

If you do this regimen consistently, you'll start to see good results after one month. If your skin begins to get red, flaky, stingy or is otherwise unhappy, see the section in chapter 1 on preventing and treating irritation from products.

Exercise and healthy eating. Exercise will improve your circulation and thus your "glow" factor. Getting the sugar, white flour and artery-clogging trans and saturated fats out of your diet and eating foods with high color in the form of fruits, veggies, and some lean protein will make you feel strong, energetic, and up for exercise. Cut the caffeine to two cups in the morning and don't forget to get seven to eight hours of sleep at night. You'll be amazed at how much better you look and feel!

Weeks 2 and 3 Goals

You'll be starting to see the results of your hard work now—so stay with it!

- Keep your weekly aesthetician appointments.
- Stay with your products.
- You'll be seeing your dermatologist for Botox and/or some filler in week two or three.
- Keep up that walking and healthy eating—if you forget or get busy, just start again the next day.

Week 4—The Finish Line

By now your skin texture and tone should be looking much improved. Your frown lines should be barely visible. The upper-lip lines and lines from your nose to your mouth or your mouth to your chin ("parentheses") should be filled with Juvederm or Restylane. The crow's feet area around your eyes should look much softer from the Botox.

This is the week when you want to go get a great haircut, make sure your hair color looks good, and maybe invest an hour in going to a department store to get a makeover—my favorites are Bobbi Brown, MAC, and Laura Mercier. Bobbi Brown's beauty book can teach you how to use makeup effectively—and often drugstore products work just fine.

Don't forget to keep up your exercise program, walking thirty minutes at least four times a week. Drink six to eight glasses of water per day, eat lots of fruits and vegetables, and fresh fish (salmon is great) at least twice a week for the entire month (if you're pregnant, though, you should avoid certain fish on your doctor's advice).

By week four you should be able to coast into your trip feeling confident in your skin. Leave a little time that week just in case you need to adjust any small problems with your Botox or Restylane (this is rarely needed). Have your last facial. Don't forget to pack your new products, especially your sunscreen, and have a fabulous time!

IN SIX MONTHS YOU COULD . . . (FOR EXAMPLE)

- improve your "glow" factor with products, peels, and microdermabrasion
- relax frown lines, crow's feet, and neck lines with Botox
- fill in the lines from your nose to your mouth and your mouth to your chin with HAs
- fill upper lip lines and improve lip contour and volume
- get some tightening and lift of the whole face with a Thermage treatment
- tighten the skin of the eyelids with an eyelid Thermage
- improve wrinkles, brown spots and acne scars with Fraxel
- get rid of brown/age spots and redness/dilated blood vessels with a series of gentle laser treatments—photorejuvenation
- remove unwanted facial hair
- clean out pores and improve acne

I HAVE SIX MONTHS

Let's pretend that in six months, you have your twenty-fifth high school or college reunion. Maybe you've been busy raising children or working in a demanding job—or both. You haven't had much time or money in the past few years for yourself. But now that's about to change—your kids are old enough to be left with a sitter or your teens are off to college, and you're finally ready to spend some time and money on yourself! A reunion gives you good motivation.

If you're over forty, realistically you'll need six months at least to repair your skin, unless you've been protecting yourself well for the last twenty years or so. A year is even better, as you'll read below, but you can accomplish a lot in six months with current technology. While the fixes you can do in one month tend to be more temporary, what you can accomplish in six begins to give you more permanent repair of sun-damaged skin. This plan is also more expensive. If you do most of the above, expect to spend about seven thousand to twelve thousand dollars—but you can also pick and choose for significantly less, say, in the range of fifteen hundred to three thousand dollars.

A six- or twelve-month plan is also much more amenable if you have a busy schedule. Most of us don't have the time or inclination to spend two or three hours a week going to appointments! So, for a six-month plan, assume that you'll need approximately two to four appointments per month, depending on your skin concerns.

Everyone has individual skin needs, so your plan will differ from someone else's and, most likely, from the plan I propose here. Keep in mind that the example here is of one type of schedule that a woman in her forties or fifties might follow for a six-month period to undertake serious repair of her sun-damaged skin. I'm also going to assume the following for this hypothetical plan:

- You're over forty.
- You have some wrinkles on your forehead, some frown lines, and some wrinkles around the eyes in the crow's feet area.

- You have some sun damage in the form of either brown spots or red spots or both.
- You have some crinkly skin around your eyelid area but don't really need an eyelid surgery.
- There's a little sagging of skin around your jawline and mouth area.
- I assume you need to go back to work and family responsibilities after treatments and cannot afford significant time off from work—that you just need to be able to cover things with makeup reasonably well.

Also keep in mind that there are different ways to get to the same goals, and that if you asked two expert dermatologists they may differ in their approach, have different lasers, or put things in a different order. That's all okay. What matters is that you find a cosmetic dermatologist who's experienced (see the regional guide in the Resources section at the back) and has a range of technology to offer you. Even two expert Botox injectors will not inject Botox exactly the same way.

A proposed six-month plan might look something like this:

Month 1 Goals

- Read the material in the first section of this chapter.
- Update your skin-care regimen to make sure that it includes at least one vitamin-A cousin (Renova, Retin-A, Tazorac, Retinol 1.0, etc.), a good antioxidant like SkinCeutical's C E Ferulic or Prevage, and a state-of-the-art sunscreen that blocks UVA as well as UVB.
- Find and make an appointment with a good cosmetic dermatologist who does laser work as well as injectables, like Botox and Restylane or Juvederm.
- Schedule your first Botox treatment to soften your crow's feet, your frown lines, and any forehead lines or prominent neck bands you might have. Schedule your follow-up treatment three to four months later if this is your first Botox.

- Schedule Restylane/Juvederm to fill the lines from your nose to your mouth and your mouth to your chin. Schedule your second treatment about a month before your event.
- Find a good aesthetician—check with your dermatologist's office first.

Month 2 Goals

- Start your photorejuvenation laser treatments to tackle any brown blotches or red blotches (see chapter 9 for details). Schedule one treatment a month for the next four to five months. If you aren't red, and you have more wrinkles and brown spots, Fraxel may be a better choice.
- Schedule and do your Thermage to tighten the skin along the jaw line, around the mouth, and give you a little lift above the eyebrows. It takes four to six months to see full results of this technology.
- Schedule and do your eyelid Thermage to tighten the crepey skin around the eyes.
- If you have unwanted facial hair, schedule four to five laser hair removal treatments about four to six weeks apart with your dermatologist.

Month 3 Goals

- Do photorejuvenation or Fraxel treatment number two. If you have a lot of brown spots, a microdermabrasion about a week to ten days after the photorejuvenation or Fraxel will help remove the brown spots that are ready to flake off.
- Do laser facial hair treatment two.

Month 4 Goals

- Do your second Botox treatment to refresh what was done in first month.

- Do photorejuvenation or Fraxel treatment number three.
- Do laser facial hair treatment three, if needed.

Month 5 Goals

- Do photorejuvenation or Fraxel treatment number four.
- Schedule your last Juvederm or Restylane treatment to fill any obvious lines or folds before your event.
- Consider CosmoPlast or CosmoDerm in your upper-lip lines (if they're a problem) about three weeks before your event. Neither last as long as Juvederm or Restylane.

Month 6—Coast into the Home Stretch

- Do your last photorejuvenation or Fraxel treatment early in the month, if needed.
- Schedule last light peel or microdermabrasion for texture improvement about ten to fourteen days before your event.

You should be ready! Your jawline should be a little tighter, your frown lines, crow's feet, upper-lip lines and lines around your mouth gone or much softer, and your skin even in color, without the brown spots and veins. You should also notice better skin texture with more "glow." You should look rested and refreshed but without that stretched look of a facelift. Have fun and enjoy that reunion!

There are many different considerations that go into putting together an individualized plan for your skin. But the above gives you an example of the kinds of services that you might want.

I HAVE NINE TO TWELVE MONTHS— TOTAL NONSURGICAL FACIAL REJUVENATION

You may read this and think, "This is exactly what I've been looking for—I can't wait to get started!" Or you may have the opposite reaction, "This is just way too much time, money, and energy, and I'm just not that

IN TWELVE MONTHS YOU COULD . . .
(FOR EXAMPLE)

- accomplish all of the six-month goals at a more relaxed pace
- improve your surface texture and your "glow" factor
- relax frown lines, crow's feet, and neck lines with Botox
- fill in the lines from your nose to your mouth and your mouth to your chin with Restylane/Juvederm
- fill upper-lip lines and improve lip contour and volume with CosmoDerm/CosmoPlast
- get some tightening and lift of the whole face with a Thermage treatment
- tighten the skin of the eyelids with an eyelid Thermage
- get rid of brown/age spots and redness/dilated blood vessels with a series of gentle laser treatments—photorejuvenation
- improve wrinkles and brown spots with fractional laser resurfacing or traditional resurfacing
- get more tightening and lift with a second Thermage treatment
- remove unwanted facial hair
- fill in hollow or sagging cheeks with Sculptra or Juvederm/Restylane
- redefine cheek bones with Sculptra and/or Restylane/Juvederm
- complete a series of treatments for acne scarring (chapter 10)
- clean out pores and improve acne

interested." Or you might want to pick and choose from the menu after prioritizing your own goals.

Some of my patients like to address one concern at a time, picking and choosing the things they want to fix about their faces. But many others really like to have a plan that clearly delineates a time frame and more ambitious goals. Some women start self-improvement with skin improvement, and tackle exercise, weight loss or diet, and nutrition all at the same time. To accomplish the twelve-month plan, you'll need approximately one to two appointments per month.

The nice thing about nonsurgical treatments is that you can go as fast or slow as you like. You can do as little or as much as you want, and you can do it with little or no time lost from your normal work activities, social activities, and family responsibilities. And, because the changes are gradual, most people can't identify a sudden change or the work you've done; they're only aware that you look better!

For the twelve-month program, particularly if you're in your sixties or seventies, you should be planning on an expense somewhere between seven thousand and sixteen thousand dollars. At that price, you're probably thinking, "Why don't I just go ahead and get a facelift?" That certainly would be an option, but remember that facelifts solve only certain problems. If it's your upper-lip lines that are bothering you, for example, or the fact that you're seeing hollowing in your cheeks, a facelift could actually make those look worse. With a nonsurgical program, you also don't face the inherent risks of surgery and anesthesia.

Month 1

- Read the material in the first section of this chapter.
- Update your skin-care regimen to make sure that it includes at least one vitamin-A cousin (Renova, Retin-A, Tazorac, Retinol 1.0, etc.), a good antioxidant like Celex C Vitamin C complex or Repenix Cream with 90 percent polyphends, and a state-of-the-art sunscreen that blocks UVA.
- Find and make an appointment with a good cosmetic dermatologist who does laser work as well as injectables.
- Schedule and do your first Botox treatment to soften your crow's feet, your frown lines, and any forehead lines or prominent neck bands you might have. Plan on four to six appointments the first year. After that, two or three appointments per year usually suffices.

- Schedule and do Restylane or Juvederm to fill the lines from your nose to your mouth and your mouth to your chin. Schedule your second treatment about four to six months later.
- Find a good aesthetician—check with your dermatologist's office first.
- Start the skin-prep process with a light peel or microdermabrasion with your aesthetician.

Months 2 and 3

- Start your Fraxel or photorejuvenation (IPL) with laser treatment number one to get rid of any brown blotches or red blotches (See chapter 9 for details). Schedule one treatment a month for the next four to five months. Choose Fraxel if you have more wrinkles and brown spots. Choose photorejuvenation if you are more red or have very few wrinkles.
- If you have a lot of brown spots, schedule a microdermabrasion about a week to ten days after the photorejuvenation. The microdermabrasion will speed the resolution of the brown/age spots.
- Or, if your problem is deep wrinkles, then now's the time to consider a traditional carbon dioxide or erbium resurfacing.
- If you have acne scarring, start your treatments soon—your dermatologist can give you a schedule of treatments.
- Schedule and do your Thermage to tighten the skin a little along the jawline, around the mouth, and give you a little lift above the eyebrows. It takes four to six months to see full results of this technology.
- Start laser treatments to remove any unwanted facial hair now—this usually takes four to six treatments to start and then maintenance once or twice a year.

Months 4 and 5

- Do your second Botox treatment.

- Do photorejuvenation or Fraxel treatments number two and number three.
- Schedule and do your eyelid Thermage to tighten the crepey skin around the eyes.
- Do laser facial hair treatments number two and number three.

Month 6

- Do photorejuvenation or Fraxel treatment number four.
- Schedule a repeat Restylane or Juvederm treatment as you had done in month one, if needed.
- If you got a good result with your first Thermage, this is the time to consider a second if you're over fifty. Do Thermage before any Sculptra.

Months 7 and 8

- If you're over forty and have a low body weight with hollowing in your cheeks, consider a series of Sculptra treatments over the next four to six months to fill that volume. If you're under forty, consider using Juvederm or Restylane to replace the volume in your cheeks or cheekbones.

Months 9 and 10

You get a break for two months!! Maybe a facial or two and relax.

Months 11 and 12

Remember to have your last treatment two to three weeks before the big event in case you bruise–a facial is fine even in that last week.

- Schedule and do a maintenance photorejuvenation appointment if you need it (it's been six months since you finished your series).
- Schedule the same for any unwanted facial hair.
- Consider CosmoPlast or CosmoDerm in your upper-lip lines, if they are a problem, about three weeks before your event.

- Do your last Botox and Juvederm or Restylane before the event.
- It's okay to schedule that last light peel or microdermabrasion for texture improvement about ten to fourteen days before the event.

Congratulations! Your skin thanks you and it looks younger, healthier, less wrinkled, more even in color and texture and has a "glow." The repair phase for your skin is done and now maintenance is much, much easier and less time consuming. Two to four appointments a year should be all you need. Enjoy your new confidence and look.

THE BOTTOM LINE

- It's possible to improve your skin a lot in a relatively short time.
- Think repair (we'll talk about maintenance later).
- Yes, it can seem expensive, but how much do you spend on vacations, restaurants, clothes, cars, even lattes every year?
- How much time do you spend *in* your skin? Probably a lot more time than in your car. People *see* you in your skin a lot more.
- How much money do you spend on products? Can you cut that back a bit and use the savings to pick and choose specific ways to improve your skin and face?
- One of the best professional rewards is to help women improve their skin, who then feel that added lift of self-confidence, which in turn ripples out into all sorts of positive effects on their families, their work, and their communities.

For more information see *surgeryfreemakeover.com.*

12

HELP ME! I'M ON A BUDGET!

Knowing your body gives you the power to change it, maintain, decorate it and strengthen it."
—You, The Owner's Manual, Mehmet Oz and Michael Roizen

I remember once spending about twenty minutes talking with a patient about her goals for her skin, the options to treat those goals, and how much things would cost. She then looked at me and said, "Oh, I can't possibly afford that." Yet before her appointment was over, she had gone on to tell me in some detail about the expensive three-week Hawaiian vacation she was just about to take. It never occurred to her that there might be a contradiction there. A luxury vacation was part of her life. But five thousand dollars on her skin seemed like a huge and unexpected outlay. It's a matter of perspective.

Everyone has different money priorities. Some have more money than others, and some people spend it in ways that seem like madness to others. Whether it's your skin, or a new car, or remodeling your house, only you can know what's best.

Given that we *do* have different money priorities and budgets, what *is* the value of improving your appearance by improving your skin? Let's start by reaffirming that your *inner* beauty will always be your greatest quality. In a *perfect* world, we would all be judged according to our character and disposition, not how we look.

In his book *Blink,* Malcolm Gladwell marshals research to show that people make almost instantaneous judgments about other people—about whether they'll be good workers, whether they'll be trustworthy, whether they're intelligent and likable. The evidence shows what we all know deep down, which is that appearances influence these judgments.

Still, as much as we might like to improve our appearance with a makeover, sometimes it's just not feasible at the moment. If the trouble is getting the bills paid, you're not going to want to spend a lot of money on your skin. Give yourself a one-hundred- or two-hundred-dollar budget and stick to that for now, postponing any major repair work for later. On the other hand, if you're spending money in other places that might go toward your surgery-free makeover, you might do the math on what you'd save, for instance, by spending less on restaurants, home remodels, postponing the new car, taking a less expensive vacation, or not spending so much on clothes.

As you read the following and develop your own budget, think in terms of repair, then maintenance. The repair phase for skin over forty (approximately), which generally lasts anywhere from six months to one year, is more time and money intensive. After that, maintenance gets much easier and much less expensive. Chapter 15 has more information on maintenance.

GETTING STARTED—I HAVE LESS THAN $1,000

If your skin is in pretty good shape, less than a thousand dollars can be enough. On the other hand, if you're fifty-five and have a lot of blotchiness, sagging, and wrinkles, you can get started with that amount. But, realistically speaking, it likely won't get you very far.

Still—get started! Think of the tortoise and the hare. A little bit over a long period gets you to the same place as a lot over a short period. I remember once reading an Ann Landers column where a woman wrote in saying that she was hesitant to go to medical school because by the time she finished her medical school training plus residency, she would be

UPDATE YOUR SKIN-CARE REGIMEN	
AM	
Cleanse with Cetaphil Gentle Skin Cleanser	$12
Replenix Cream, an antioxident	$54
Cetaphil Moisturizer with SPF 15 or Oil of Olay Regenerist SPF 15	$15–18
PM	
Cleanse with Cetaphil Gentle Skin Cleanser	See above
Apply SkinMedica Retinol Complex	$50
Cetaphil Moisturizing Lotion or Cream	$10
Peels or microdermabrasion	
Light peel	$60
or microdermabrasion with an aesthetician preferably employed by your dermatologist's office	$125
Botox on a budget	
Just pick either your frown lines or your crow's feet, whichever is worse	$400
Update your makeup	
Here are five products to give you a good bang for your buck:	
Laura Mercier Special Concealer	$22
Laura Mercier Tinted Moisturizer SPF 15 or the Jane Iredale Powder Foundation SPF 18	$40–48
Lancôme Définicils Mascara in black	$23
Dior Eyeliner Pencil	$24
Bobbi Brown's SPF 15 lip shine	$19
GRAND TOTAL	**$775–851**

seven years older and almost forty years old. Ann Landers replied with the question, "How old will you be in seven years if you don't go to medical school?"

If you have less than a thousand dollars to spend, focus on these four things:

- improving your daily skin care program with products
- inexpensive peels and microdermabrasion
- Botox on a budget or Juvederm or Restylane
- great makeup options

What follows is a sample plan with a budget for one of my patients. Again, this is a real person, and everyone is different. So don't go out and copy this verbatim. This is meant to be an example of how you could go about preparing this type of program for your skin on a budget. All costs are approximate and product availability can change. For online information go to *www.skintour.com.*

You can see that for not a whole lot of money, you can make a pretty significant difference in your skin. If you can afford it, I would vote for doing the microdermabrasion or light peels once every four to eight weeks. The skin-care products should last two to four months for each of the above. For maintenance, the Botox will need to be repeated three times the first year (this depends on your age and the strength of the muscles). But as the muscles relax, many women can go every five or six months after a year or so.

GETTING STARTED—I HAVE $3,000 OR LESS

For a little more, three thousand dollars or less, you can add some laser treatments for brown spots or red spots, or an allover face tightening with Thermage, more Botox, or fillers like Restylane or Juvederm.

Remember, this example is a skin program for a real person. Your skin plan will be different, and again, all costs are approximate and product availability may change.

A Better Skin-Care Program

A great skin-care program should include a gentle cleanser, a good moisturizer, a sunscreen that blocks UVA well, a vitamin-A cream (Renova,
Retinol 1.0, Retin-A, Tazorac, etc.), an antioxidant serum or cream, an eye
cream, and a gentle scrub. A possible skin-care program in this range
might look like this:

BETTER SKIN-CARE PROGRAM	
AM	
Cetaphil Gentle Skin Cleanser	$12
Prevage or SkinCeuticals C E Ferrulic (antioxidant)	$100–128
MD Forte Replenish Hydrating Cream (or any other moisturizer you love and only if needed)	$40
SkinMedica Envrionmental Defense Sunscreen SPF 30 (moisturizing sunscreen) or La Roche-Posay Anthelios SPF 30	$30
Dermalogica Total Eyecare (with SPF 15)	$32
PM	
Cetaphil Gentle Skin Cleanser	
MD Forte Replenish Hydrating Cream (or any other moisturizer you love) then wait 15 minutes	
Renova (prescription) or Cellex-C Retional Complex (vitamin A cream)	$50–125
Elizabeth Arden Eye Cream	$40
Once or twice a week	
Use your gentle scrub (I like the Bobbi Brown Skin Refining Cream)	$50
PRODUCT TOTAL	**$364–467**

Botox.   Depending on what you'd like done, with a little extra money you can treat more than just one area. For example, you might want to inject your frown lines and your crow's feet areas. If you have prominent horizontal forehead lines or problems in your lower face, you can tackle those areas as well. Costs vary by your age and your region.

Botox	$600–800

Fillers.   In this price range, I would recommend still sticking with the hyaluronic acid fillers like Restylane and Juvederm. Most of the time you would need your filler treatments only twice a year. Consider using two or three syringes. With the extra syringe you could fix those "parentheses" lines, but you could also add a little fullness to your lips, fill in lost volume in the chin area and at the jawline, or put a little Restylane or Juvederm in your frown lines. If you have very deep folds from your nose to your mouth and heavier cheeks, you may need two syringes in that area alone.

Fillers—one syringe	$500

Photorejuvenation and Thermage.   Since you are budgeting three thousand dollars or less to get started, you can't spend money on both Botox and fillers and still have two thousand to twenty-five hundred dollars left for laser treatments. You'll need to make a choice between Botox and fillers or photorejuvenation and Thermage.

I would recommend staying away from the fractional resurfacing devices, like Fraxel, in this price range. A series of Fraxel treatments will run from three thousand to five thousand dollars, which would put you outside your budget. Thermage or photorejuvenation (about two thousand to twenty-five hundred dollars), on the other hand, would be possible.

Series of photorejuvenation treatments for color problems	$2,500
or Full-face Thermage for skin tightening	$2,500
TOTAL	$2,500

You can see that with three thousand dollars or under you can make a significant improvement in your skin and, although you may not be able to do everything that you want, you can target your main problem areas and focus on those. If your problem is mostly wrinkles, for example, choose the Botox and fillers. If the problem is mostly sagging along your jawline, then Thermage may just do the trick. Or, a series of photorejuvenation laser treatments to remove brown spots and red spots or blood vessels may be your first priority. You won't be able to do all of the above with this amount, but you can certainly get a good start toward your goals. There's really no rush, and a little bit over a long period still gets you to your goal—remember the tortoise.

$5,000 AND UP—MONEY IS NOT AN ISSUE: TOTAL NONSURGICAL FACIAL REJUVENATION— GETTING STARTED

If you're at a point in your life where money is no object, that brings some blessings but also some problems. With so many choices in skin care products—literally thousands of products at this point—and the explosion of new technology involving fillers, lasers and radiofrequency waves (and combinations of them all), it can be very difficult to evaluate what works and what doesn't. Add to that all the marketing dollars spent by skin-care and skin-device companies and the confusion escalates almost exponentially.

You might think, "Well, why not just do everything?" But you risk wasting a lot of time (and money), and any procedure can have complications—why risk those unnecessarily?

A Luxury Skin-Care Program

If money is no object, you might want to try some of the luxury brands with exotic ingredients (all unproven) to see if they work for you. When you change products, change one at a time so that you will know which one is the culprit if you get irritated or have an allergic reaction. Use a product for three to six months before you decide that it's delivering on its promises.

With an unlimited budget, it is possible to try the exotic and the unusual alike:

- Revive Intensive Volumizing Serum—$600 for one ounce—contains epidermal growth factor
- Sisley Paris Sisleya Elixir—$390 for less than one ounce—contains extracts of weeping willow, gingko biloba, and something "marine"
- Cle de Peau Beaute La Crème—$475 for one ounce
- Dermagenetics DNA Test & Custom Anti-Wrinkle Night Cream—$400 for one ounce—purports to make a custom cream for you based on a swab of cells from inside your mouth
- Natura Bisse Inhibit-Dermafill—$385 for one ounce—contains 40 percent octapeptide
- Kanebo Sensai Ex La Crème—$368 for 1.36 ounces—silk derivatives, apricot kernal extracts, and hyaluonate
- Darphin Replenishing Anti-Wrinkle Serum—$310 for one ounce—horsetail extract, iris extract, and vital essence of "mamaku"

You're now asking, are these worth the money? No one knows. There is no reliable research on any of them.

Below is a luxury skin plan for a real person. While your personal skin plan will vary, the plan below will give you some idea of how you might go about preparing a similar program for your skin. All costs are approximate and product availability can change.

A luxury skin-care program should still include the basics: a gentle cleanser, a good moisturizer, a sunscreen that blocks UVA well, a vitamin-A cream (Renova, Retinol 1.0, Retin-A, Tazorac, etc.), an antioxidant serum or cream, an eye cream, and a gentle scrub. A possible skin-care program in this range might look like this:

LUXURY SKIN-CARE PROGRAM	
AM	
Éminence Organic Lemon Cleanser	$38
TNS Recovery Cream (cell growth factors)	$140
Crème de la Mer (or any other moisturizer you love and only if needed)	$130
SkinMedica Environmental Defense Sunscreen (moisturizing sunscreen) or La Roche-Posay Anthelios SPF 30	$30
Colorescience My Favorite Eye Cream (with 22 percent zinc for sunscreen)	$25
PM	
Éminence Organic Lemon Cleanser	
Crème de la Mer (or any other moisturizer you love and only if needed)	
Renova (prescription) or SkinMedica Retinol Complex (vitamin A cream) use the Renova and Vitamin C on alternate nights	$50–125
SkinCeuticals C E Ferrulic (antioxidant)	$115–128
SkinCeuticals Eye Balm	$70
Once or twice a week	
Use your gentle scrub (I like the Bobbi Brown Skin Refining Cream)	$50
PRODUCT TOTAL	**$648–736**

Add to this one of the luxury products above if you like.

Botox.   Depending on your face, you can treat more than just one area. For example, you might want to address your frown lines and crow's feet area. If you have prominent horizontal forehead lines or problems in your lower face, you can tackle those areas as well. It's important if you're using more Botox to make sure your injector is an expert injector. Experts only, please, for the lower face.

Botox	$600–1,000

Fillers.   In this price range, I would recommend still sticking with the hyaluronic-acid fillers like Restylane and Juvederm. Instead of budgeting for just one syringe, you can use as many as needed. Most of the time you would need your filler treatments only twice a year. With the extra syringes you could do the lines from your nose to your mouth and from your mouth to your chin. You could also fill in some of the loss of volume in the chin area itself, including that little notch that so many of us get between the chin and the cheek right along the jawline. You might also be able to put a little Restylane in your frown lines. If you have very deep folds from your nose to your mouth and heavier cheeks, you may need two syringes in that area alone. You could also decide that you wanted to see how a little cheek augmentation would look. Generally, that takes about one syringe per cheek.

Sculptra to fill out hollow cheeks or the lower face is an option in this price range. An initial series of treatments, depending on how much product you need, would be three thousand to ten thousand dollars. This seems like a lot but Sculptra is the only product I've seen where an expert dermatologist or plastic surgeon can achieve an almost facelift-like effect nonsurgically. Maintenance is minimal—usually one treatment every twelve to twenty-four months. Sculptra is approved in Canada and Europe for all uses. It is FDA approved in the United States for HIV patients, but full approval is pending in 2008. Other uses are currently "off-label."

Fillers	$1000–10,000

Photorejuvenation and Thermage. If you are fairly wrinkle-free but you have slight sagging along the jawline and redness or brown blotchiness, then you should consider Thermage skin tightening and a series of gentle laser photorejuvenation. These would tighten that sagging skin along the jawline and remove or reduce the redness or brown spots. If you have wrinkles, you may want to consider a fractional laser series. For example

Series of photorejuvenation treatments for color problems	$2,500
Full-face Thermage for skin tightening	$2,500
or Fraxel laser—series of 5	$5,000

THINKING ABOUT YOUR SKIN PLAN'S BUDGET

Each generation defines aging differently from the one before. My grandmother's generation, for instance, had different expectations than my mother's. Our generation certainly has very different expectations for the aging process than our mothers! Sure, natural and intrinsic aging occurs. We all know that. But there's a big difference between a great-looking, healthy fifty-five-year-old and a fifty-five-year-old whose skin is leathery and sun-damaged, and who is out of shape and not in good health. Those are two extremes, of course. But much of what happens in between those extremes really *is* affected by all the daily things that we do to promote our skin health and our general health. I think it's worth spending some

LASERS

How can you sort out which lasers work and are worth spending your money on? The answer to this is that by yourself, you probably can't. You'll need expert help, and even that at times is tough.

Laser systems. In the early to mid-1990s, two main laser companies produced about six or seven types of lasers. Now dozens of laser companies make anywhere from three to ten laser systems *each,* creating a market overflowing with more than a hundred lasers, all clamoring for attention. The last decade or so has also seen a tremendous change in the ways lasers are sold to doctors. Originally, laser companies tested their lasers themselves for long periods of time before releasing them to the world at large. Their very reputation depended on delivering a safe and reliable device that got good results for patients.

But due to the more intense competition now, laser companies all vie to be the first to get to market with their new devices, each with their "new" technology. And while this "new" technology may be promising, lasers are often released before the results are clearly defined and before the treatment parameters are definitively established. That means, all too often, that doctors and consumers do the "testing" of the devices themselves.

Doctors and patients need to beware. With such a wide variety of lasers being used on so many people, it may be several years before any problems and complications of particular devices come to the attention of an individual company, consumers, and doctors.

money, care, and time on our skin to go into our fifties, sixties, seventies, eighties, and maybe nineties, feeling good about our physical selves.

However, only you can decide if the money spent on something is worth the price. No one should ever go into financial debt to improve her skin. Instead, take a look at your budget, your goals, and review with your dermatologist what seems like a feasible and affordable skin plan to get your glowing skin back!

THE BOTTOM LINE

- You can make a difference in your skin for less money than you think.
- Daily habits really matter and can be inexpensive.
- Read through the chapters in this book on your problem areas to pinpoint your priorities and get a sense for the benefits and risks of different treatments.
- You can sometimes spread out your treatments to accommodate your budget—you may be able get to the same place doing a few things over a year or two years versus a lot in nine months.
- Prioritize your trouble areas and spend money on those first.
- Having an unlimited budget is great, but be careful whom you choose to work with.
- Remember the maintenance phase is much less expensive then the repair phase if you have many problems to fix.

PART FIVE

FOCUS ON LIFESTYLE AND YOUR SKIN'S HEALTH

13

THE FOOD, LIFESTYLE, AND SKIN CONNECTION

Skin, just like any other organ in our body, is only as healthy as the rest of us. It becomes unhealthy if we smoke, eat junk food, drink too much alcohol, and become couch potatoes. That's why it's almost impossible (unless you're sixteen years old) to have beautiful skin if you aren't paying attention to food and lifestyle issues. If you want beautiful skin, this chapter outlines the basic things to do to get it. These steps may seem very simple, but that's the whole idea: to give you a short list of items that are easy to remember and integrate into your daily routines. There's no hard-to-follow diet here or radical lifestyle-change recommendations.

FOUR QUICK DIETARY CHANGES YOU CAN MAKE TO IMPROVE YOUR SKIN

1. ***Eat at least six foods with color a day.*** Color means bright colors, and bright colors mean foods rich in antioxidants, flavonoids, plant-based cancer-fighting compounds, and fiber. Another plus to eating colorful foods is that they'll likely fill you up sooner—a good thing if you're looking to shave off a few pounds or maintain a normal weight.

211

Strive to include two or three foods with bright colors at every meal. For example, at breakfast that might mean adding a few blueberries to your cereal and drinking a glass of orange juice with pulp (with calcium). For lunch it might mean a salad, which usually contains two or three other veggies besides lettuce. A sandwich that has lettuce, tomato, and onion also counts. At dinner you might try a curry with two or three different vegetables or have a green, yellow, or red vegetable plus a small salad with your protein source. Get creative! Broiling a half tomato with grated parmesan and little garlic olive oil drizzled on it is easy and takes five to ten minutes. Bake a couple of yams for an hour while you watch your favorite show and then mash them the next night with ginger and a little maple syrup. Fabulous and fast!

You get the idea. There are many delicious ways to get those health-building delicious vegetables that come in such variety and abundance. Most Americans eat a very small range of the options available to them.

2. *Eat more fish and foods high in "good fats."* By now, everyone knows not to touch trans fats (partially hydrogenated oils) unless your goal is to clog most of the small and large arteries in your body. You have to read labels to avoid these. Look for the terms *partially hydrogenated oils* or *trans fats* on the label. Eating these trans fats is like putting glue into your blood vessels.

Also keep your saturated fats low. These are the fats that make blood vessel walls sticky, causing plaque to build up inside them. This, over time, thickens the walls, which decreases the amount of room there is for what we really need—blood. Your skin is no exception—it looks better when your circulation is good.

The goal is to keep all of your blood vessels as wide open as possible to permit as much blood flow as you can, but also to keep them flexible. So what does fish have to do with all this? Healthy oils help to preserve the health of your blood vessels and may even help to reverse some of the damage done by trans fats and the over-consumption of saturated fats. Fish, particularly ones like salmon, are high in the good types of fat as are olive oil and some other plant-based oils like safflower oil. And these oils are some of the building blocks of the natural oils in your skin that help to keep skin flexible. Eat one to three servings of fish per week (unless you're pregnant; in which case, be sure to get a list of "safe" fish and the healthy amounts to eat from your obstetrician). Even if you're not pregnant, pay attention to the "safe" fish lists. Fish can contain various carcinogens and health-sapping heavy metals like mercury. Some "farmed" fish are safe and some, particularly those farmed in China, are not.

3. *Eat less sugar.*   I'm not a sugar Nazi, but the large amount of sugar in our diets is not good for us for a multitude of reasons. There is evidence that sugar "glycosylates" our cells' proteins, which contributes to accelerated aging. Simply put, the sugar molecules attach to our cells' proteins, keeping them from doing their jobs efficiently. This affects all the organs in our body, including the skin. Sugar is just empty calories with no nutrition. Eating sugars, particularly on an empty stomach, also stresses your pancreas, which then has to pump out huge amounts of insulin to compensate for all the sugar. Avoid sugary drinks, baked goods (unless they are whole grain), and candy in particular.

4. *Drink plenty of water (sodas don't count).*   Most of us know we should drink four to eight glasses of water a day, and yet many of us still don't. Keep your own water bottle handy during the day, or get a Brita filter and keep it near your desk or kitchen counter.

SIX SIMPLE LIFESTYLE CHANGES TO MAKE YOUR SKIN GLOW

1. *Sleep seven to nine hours a night.*   Most of us need seven to nine hours of sleep to function optimally, and that includes our skin. We all know someone somewhere—an old college friend, coworker, fellow athlete—who seems to do just fine on four or five hours a night. And, we all probably wish we were that person. But let's face it, 99 percent of us are *not* that person.

Your skin will tell you immediately when you are not getting enough sleep. You know it yourself. You look tired, your skin looks gray, you look haggard and unhealthy—particularly if that lack of sleep was preceded by a night of too much alcohol.

Roizen and Oz, the authors of *You: The Owner's Manual,* say that getting a minimum of seven hours of sleep per night adds about three years to your lifespan. They also point out that fatigue lowers our ability to make good choices in all sorts of different situations.

2.   ***Limit alcohol and coffee consumption to moderate doses.***   Coffee is a great drug, and caffeine-containing compounds have been used for centuries across a wide variety of different cultures. Like most drugs, though, just because a small amount is good doesn't mean that a lot is better. In fact, the reverse is almost always true for anything that doesn't naturally occur inside our body.

A cup or two a day has been shown to improve our mental functioning. More than that interferes with our sleep and can make us overstimulated and jittery. Drinking too much coffee also has a negative effect on our bodies' absorption of calcium—calcium being something most of us don't get enough of in the first place. If you have rosacea (a skin disease characterized by flushing and broken blood vessels on the face), too much coffee will aggravate it.

As for alcohol, a little bit has been shown to make us less susceptible to heart problems. But too much is dehydrating and toxic to our organs—and dehydration is death for our skin (just think of the way you look after a night of too much alcohol and not enough sleep, and you'll get the picture). How much is too much? For the average-sized (non-pregnant) woman, one drink per day on average is the maximum for good health. For a male, two drinks per day on average is the maximum allowed. It doesn't count to have five drinks over the course of one night; it's the daily intake of a *small amount* of alcohol that has health benefits, not loading up on one or two days of the week.

3.   ***Exercise four to five days a week.***   My primary care doctor, Dr. Bliss, a fabulous internist, calls exercise the "fountain of youth." If you need to convince yourself of this, just look around.

Pick any three people you know who are in their sixties. Try to pick at least one person who has exercised regularly for at least twenty years and compare the shape they are in, their general sense of energy, their youthful appearance, their weight, and so forth, to the person who doesn't exercise. By age sixty, there's a big difference between people who exercise regularly and people who don't.

So how does exercise help your skin? Like with every other organ, exercise dilates the blood vessels and gets the blood moving vigorously through the skin, which carries away waste and brings life-building, fresh oxygen. The other benefits of exercise include helping to preserve bone strength, building and protecting the heart muscle, helping to control blood pressure, aiding in mental health and stress reduction, helping to prevent obesity, and building strength. What's not to like?

The best exercise programs build on something you like to do. Combine some cardiovascular aerobic training (like running, cycling, swimming) with strength-building exercises (like weights, some yoga, some Pilates), flexibility maintenance (stretching, yoga, Pilates), balance training, which is very important as we get older (yoga poses on one foot, balance balls or bosu balls, dance), and endurance (walking, hiking, longer bicycle rides, distance running).

Many exercise programs contain one or two of these but do not contain all of them. Be sure as you get older that you strive for a variety incorporating some of all five of these areas into your exercise program.

4. *Wear sun-protective clothing.* Using sun-protective clothing is much easier than remembering to apply sunscreen all the time. The best clothes have an SPF rating. Other clothing works to block the sun as well, but if you hold the clothing up to the light and can see right through it, you're not getting much sun protection.

5. *Have your Vitamin-D level checked.* Yes, checked! Ask to have a blood test done for it at your next doctor's appointment. It's shocking how many people in this country are deficient. You can take all the calcium in the world for your bones and it won't do you much good if you

are vitamin D deficient. This vitamin is essential for bone strength and may have anticancer effects as well.

6. ***Decrease stress.***   A wake-up call for me was when my cardiologist friend told me that chronic stress is as bad for my heart as smoking a pack a day. It turns out that our bodies are wired for stress that is periodic and intermittent. It's the same physiologic mechanism that allows us to run quickly away from danger, respond appropriately to emergencies, or find that last bit of energy to finish a marathon. Responses to this kind of stress help us to survive.

Chronic stress is a different matter, however. Chronic stress is that day-to-day stress that we all have experienced. It might be a difficult boss you have to deal with every day, a frustrating, unpredictable commute, constant financial worries, or the stress from a bad marriage. These kinds of day-to-day stress that are cumulative over many years take years off our lives and affect our skin.

Many of us have had the experience of seeing friends go through a year or two of very difficult life changes only to see them "age in front of our eyes." Perhaps it's the constant circulating of "stress hormones" that over time constricts the blood vessels supplying our skin; maybe it's inflammatory factors that are secreted when we're stressed that begin to take a toll on our faces.

Whatever our sources of chronic stress, it's clear that our health will be better if we find a way to resolve once and for all those issues that keep us from being relaxed and happy. Easier said than done, I realize, but there are plenty of ways to start working toward a stress-free life. You might, for instance, decide to see a counselor (don't be afraid to ask for help), talk to trusted friends or a clergyman/woman, or take up yoga, which can be very calming and centering. If you're not keen on organized exercise, why not try taking some long walks so you have time to think, to decompress?

7. ***Stop smoking!***   Smoking robs your skin of much-needed oxygen. It's partly the circulation in your skin that gives it its youthful glow and if you decrease oxygen levels and increase levels of carbon dioxide,

not to mention the harmful chemicals in cigarettes, blood flow to the skin decreases. Many smokers have that grayish-yellow tone to their skin in addition to many more wrinkles, particularly on the upper lip—those "smoker's lines."

THE BOTTOM LINE

- Lifestyle and dietary changes can make a big difference—instantly and over time.
- Reduce chronic stress.
- Eat plenty of foods with loads of color—the more the better.
- Control coffee and alcohol; drink plenty of water.
- Avoid artery-clogging trans and saturated fats.
- Exercise!—your skin will thank you.
- Get seven to nine hours of sleep a night.
- Use sun-protective clothing.
- Stop smoking, if you haven't already.

MENOPAUSE AND YOUR SKIN

These aren't hot flushes. They're power surges.
—*Anonymous*

Most women experience menopause—and its accompanying hot flashes—in their late forties to early fifties. Menopause can bring some frustrating new issues for your skin, or even bad flashbacks to your teen years with problems like acne. But take heart—there are good changes that come with menopause, too. Oil production decreases after menopause, which gets rid of acne (eventually) and helps shrink pore size. Your skin is more consistent and not subject to premenopausal fluctuation. Many wrinkles can be prevented and treated with good topicals, good nutrition, and modern technology. And you've never had more confidence and self-acceptance of your own beauty, because you're wiser and more comfortable with who you are!

Here are some of the concerns I hear:

- "I have acne again—what can I do?"
- "I woke up one morning with all these wrinkles just overnight."
- "My skin seems to be getting thinner."
- "I'm a little red anyway, but since these hot flashes started, I'm *really* red and it's starting to bother me."

Let's sort out the myths versus the facts.

SKIN CHANGES AS HORMONES CHANGE AT MENOPAUSE

How menopause changes our skin. At menopause and with age, our skin starts to produce less collagen and elastic fibers. Collagen is the supportive protein structure of the skin, and elastic fibers provide the ability to bounce back. So the drop in collagen and elastic fibers accelerates wrinkling and sagging.

For many years, estrogen replacement (also known as hormone replacement therapy or HRT) after menopause was common, and it helped skin retain more collagen. Then, starting in 2002 with the women's health initiative findings, HRT was suspected of increasing breast cancer risks in some women, in addition to the already known risk of uterine cancer. The correlation between HRT and breast cancer is even stronger today, and it's fair to say that HRT is being prescribed less and for shorter periods of time.

What about the effects of estrogen on skin? A 1997 study of 3,875 postmenopausal women concluded that estrogen helped older women to have younger-looking skin and that estrogen helped maintain their skin's collagen, its thickness, its elasticity, and its ability to maintain moisture. The study also found that the chances of having dry and wrinkled skin was 30 percent less in women who took estrogen replacements (HRT) in comparison with women who did not.

Another recent skin study of ninety-eight postmenopausal women with hormone-replacement therapy (gel or patches) showed increased skin thickness, skin hydration, and skin surface lipids (good fats). The study found that estrogen therapy increased the skin's thickness 7 to 15 percent and skin oil (sebum) by 35 percent.

All that said, no one should be taking HRT solely to have younger-looking skin! You'll want to talk with your primary care doctor and gynecologist about whether hormone replacement therapy is right for you and what your personal risk factors might be—and, should you decide to

TERMS YOU'LL WANT TO KNOW

- *estrogen:* maintains the uterine lining before menopause and falls by about 90 percent at menopause. Estrogens are a group of hormones, not just one.
- *progesterone:* matures the lining of the uterus in preparation for pregnancy and sloughs it off if there is no pregnancy. It also decreases about 90 percent after menopause.
- *androgens:* "male" hormones—all women have androgens, too. The main ones are testosterone and a hormone called DHEA. Androgens stay about the same or decrease slightly after menopause, but their effects are more obvious because there is less estrogen and progesterone around.

use it, what different types of hormone replacement therapy would be best for you. "Bioidentical" hormones still contain estrogen and have the disadvantage of containing variable and often unknown doses of it.

Estrogen creams on facial skin. There is almost no research on using estrogen creams or plant-based estrogenic creams directly on the facial skin, though they can be found in every pharmacy and on the shelves of natural food stores and co-ops. Until we know if they help, and how much, if anything, is absorbed into our bloodstreams from estrogen creams, it is *not* reasonable to assume these are safe. Try creams with soy which may have an estrogen-like effect.

Selective Estrogen Receptor Modulators. There may be hope in new medications called selective estrogen receptor modulators (SERMs). These SERMs can mimic the effects of estrogen in some tissues, like the skin, while inhibiting effects in others. The medical community hopes that these SERMs will allow women to take advantage of estrogen's possible benefits, such as its value in staving off osteoporosis and improving

BODY AREAS THAT MAY BE AFFECTED BY MENOPAUSE

- skin—somewhat thinner, dryer, more wrinkled
- vaginal skin—thinner, sometimes a little itchy or burning sensation, discomfort with sex
- breast tissue—glandular tissue is replaced by fatty tissue, some sagging
- bones—decreased bone calcium renders bones more brittle and prone to fractures

skin health and appearance, while reducing its risks for certain cancers. Some of the plant estrogens may work this way already. As they are studied more, we may find that certain plant estrogens have a very beneficial effect on skin while having almost no effect on breast tissue. This research may allow us to take advantage of estrogens in the future in a different, less risky way.

KEEP SKIN GLOWING AFTER MENOPAUSE

There are other ways can you build collagen and elastic fibers to keep your skin looking youthful!

Creams that build collagen.   Anything that builds collagen in your skin will help to maintain that youthful thickness, glow, and reflectivity. Retinol, Renova, Tazorac, Retin-A, and tretinon are all names for prescription vitamin-A creams. These are still the gold standard for collagen-building creams in the skin. We have twenty years of good data and millions of satisfied patients to support using these vitamin-A cousins, also called retinoids. There is also evidence to support using good-quality vitamin-C serums (Like SkinCeuticals Vitamin C E Ferrulic, Cellex-C, or Waimea Vitamin C Serum) to build collagen. Alpha- and beta-hydroxy acids are known to build collagen as well.

Scrubs.   Creams that help to shed the outer, dead layer of the skin build collagen because they send a signal to the deeper layers of the skin to become more active. These are gentle scrubs, and there are many good ones on the market. Try Bobbi Brown's Skin Refining Cream. Don't overdo these, though, particularly if you have sensitive skin. Twice a week is fine. If you have very tough, oily skin, a gentle scrub daily may be okay.

Injectables that build collagen.   The only injectable that really builds collagen currently is Sculptra. (See chapter 6 for more detail on what Sculptra is and how it works.) Sculptra is a different form of lactic acid our muscles naturally produce. When injected, Sculptra sends a signal to the cells that make collagen to make more of it. Gradually the Sculptra is absorbed by the body, just like lactic acid in our muscles. Patients end up with more collagen and more youthful skin.

Lasers that build collagen.   Carbon dioxide and erbium resurfacing lasers build collagen but are also the riskiest and have the most downtime. Fractional resurfacing lasers like the Fraxel also build collagen but with less risk and downtime. Results are good but not as good as a traditional resurfacing laser. "Long-wave" lasers (Smoothbeam, Cooltouch, Aramis) and photorejuvenation with IPLs are also known to build collagen. They send a signal to the skin to make more collagen. These are not dramatic but every little bit helps. Five monthly treatments should give you results, followed by once or twice a year for maintenance. Used over many years, they can help to maintain your skin's youthful appearance.

ACNE DURING MENOPAUSE

When many of us were teenagers, we dreamed of the day when we would be grown women and our acne gone. But time and menopause can play a trick on us.

While menopause occurs for most women in their early fifties, changes in our hormones start years earlier. Thus you may hear your doctor refer to "perimenopause," which means the months and years before actual menopause. During perimenopause, our hormonal systems are already beginning to change, even though we're still having regular periods.

Here's why this matters: acne is a hormonal disease. Beginning in puberty, hormones turn "on" our oil glands. Once the oil glands are on, they can get plugged up, the oil can harden, pores can enlarge, and bacteria can grow. And presto, you have a pimple. Without active oil glands, none of this happens—think of the blemish-free skin of a child. So some women have acne in their teens that resolves in their twenties and thirties, only to have it recur as perimenopausal hormone changes occur.

Perimenopausal acne is different from acne in the teens. Here's what's different:

- Small, tender bumps. There are fewer blackheads than whiteheads and more of what one of my patients calls "undergrounders." These small, tender cysts are most often found around the jawline, around the mouth, and sometimes on the neck.
- Less T-zone acne. There's less acne in the T-zone and the cheek area and more acne around the chin, mouth, and upper neck.
- Cysts last. The lesions last longer, sometimes taking two to four weeks to resolve rather than a few days to a week.
- Unpredictability. Sometimes menopausal women will be clear for months and then suddenly break out again.

Because acne is different in perimenopause, many of the medications, both oral and in a cream form, made for teenage acne don't work very well in perimenopausal women. Here's why:

Most acne medications are for teenage skin. Medications for teenagers are formulated for the very oily skin of that age group. Most of the time, they are much too drying for the skin of women over forty. This shows up as redness and irritation. Many of you have heard of using Renova for wrinkles but don't know it was originally made for acne in teens in the form of Retin-A. Both have antiaging, antiwrinkle effects, but both also help acne by unclogging pores and preventing clogs (comedones) from forming in the first place. Renova is better for menopausal skin because it is formulated in a moisturizing base that is made specifically for older skin. If you are trying to use Retin-A gel or cream or, for example, Tazarac gel or cream, these can be irritating because they were put in a base for teenage skin.

The acne is deeper and not superficial.   Creams, gels, and lotions that are put on the skin work well for blackheads, whiteheads and small pimples but do little for the deeper cystic-type acne that goes along with the changing hormones in the perimenopausal woman. If you do have blackheads and whiteheads, the Renova .02 percent cream will help remove those, while also preventing wrinkles and reversing sun damage— an added bonus!

Oral contraceptives.   We dermatologists will often recommend an oral medication, like an oral contraceptive, for a younger woman with acne. Because the risk of blood clots increases significantly after the age of 35 and particularly in smokers, this is not a good option for most women in their forties and fifties. Women over thirty-five shouldn't be on oral contraceptives except when recommended by a gynecologist.

Oral antibiotics.   Many dermatologists, including myself, are avoiding oral antibiotics for long periods unless they are absolutely necessary. When oral antibiotics are used too freely in conditions where they are not absolutely needed, bacteria can become resistant. For example, most people now know that trying to treat a common cold, which is caused by a virus, with an antibiotic is not helpful at all and just breeds bacterial resistance.

Also, oral antibiotics can change the "good bacteria" in our intestinal tracts, mouth, and vaginal area. This can lead to the overgrowth of yeasts and "bad bacteria." But, if necessary, oral antibiotics can work well. It's fine to use antibiotics for acne for a month or two to control a severe flare. Since it takes prescription creams and lotions eight to ten weeks to kick in, an oral antibiotic will control your acne while the topicals have a chance to start working.

What works for perimenopausal acne.   First of all, definitely consider prescription creams like Renova .02 percent cream, especially if you have a tendency toward blackheads and whiteheads. Again, you get a bonus with this in that it helps to treat wrinkles and sun damage as well as helps prevent acne. If you have a lot of those deeper cysts, particularly on the jaw line, Renova won't do much.

Spironolactone/aldactone.   This prescription medication has been around for more that thirty years and was originally used to treat kidney patients and high blood pressure. But it is very effective in low doses for treating acne. It works by reducing androgens, which are the "male" hormones that are also present in women.

How spironolactone works.   In perimenopause, the amount of androgen stays about the same. But because estrogen and progesterone are decreasing, the "male" hormones are relatively higher than they were. This can cause breakouts. Spironolactone helps control that imbalance of male and female hormones. It can also reduce facial hair growth and control PMS-type symptoms as well.

Don't take spironolactone if you have low blood pressure, because you may get dizzy. This won't happen for women with normal or slightly elevated blood pressure—lower blood pressure is a positive side effect. Also, don't take it if you are pregnant. Remember, it *is possible* to get pregnant in the perimenopausal period if you are not using birth control and are sexually active. If you are not actively preventing pregnancy, spironolactone is not for you because it could affect the development of a male fetus's genitals.

Otherwise, it is safe and has been around for many years. In low doses, it may help not only to reduce acne, facial hair growth, but also lower blood pressure a bit and prevent fluid retention with PMS.

Lasers for acne.   There are two main types of laser systems being used to treat acne. Long-wave lasers and the blue- and red-light systems.

I think it's fair to say that the protocols for treating acne with these lasers are still evolving—some people get a great result and others get fewer results than we would hope for. This is an evolving area, though, and treatments will improve over the next five to ten years. Pricing varies for these lasers so ask for an estimate at your consultation.

With the long-wave lasers, patients usually undergo a series of four or five treatments. If you see significant improvement after a short series, don't expect it to last forever: you'll need maintenance treatments two to four times a year. Examples of these lasers are the Smoothbeam, CoolTouch, the Aramis, and others. Lasers are often used in conjunction with other acne treatments, like Retin-A or Renova.

The other form of laser treatment for acne is often called Blu-U or sometimes referred to as photodynamic therapy. A clear liquid is painted on the skin and is left on for thirty to sixty minutes. Then a light is used to activate the clear liquid. In some systems, a blue light (thus the Blu-U) or red light is used, and in the other system, an IPL-type laser is used to activate the liquid.

The downside to these blue- and red-light treatments is that there is sometimes redness and peeling for three to ten days, which is similar to the peeling you might expect after a sunburn. Be prepared for some inconvenience if you sign up for this type of laser.

REAL-WORLD ADVICE

I really don't like taking anything oral but have pretty bad acne. I'm forty-five. What would you advise?   Consider a laser for acne then. If there is a good dermatologist with a laser center near you, a short series followed by maintenance should help. Expect a 50 to 80 percent reduction. Nothing is perfect for acne. Pricing really varies, so I hesitate to guess without knowing your region or the type of laser.

Would peels help my acne?   If you have blackheads and whiteheads—in other words—clogged pores—then yes. If your acne is mostly those deeper, slightly tender bumps, not as much.

Help! I'm fifty-two and still really, really oily with some clogged pores and acne.   It doesn't seem fair, does it? Acne, oil, and probably a few wrinkles at the same time. Try some of the more drying products like

Neutrogena Acne Wash, oil blotting papers, and Retin-A gel. Microdermabrasion once a month can help keep your pores cleaned out and may dry you a little. Consider a laser series or Blu-U acne treatment mentioned above or spironolactone (prescription)—both through your dermatologist. The nice thing about oily skin is that it usually doesn't wrinkle as much.

THE BOTTOM LINE

- Do everything you can to preserve and maintain your collagen and elastic fibers.
- Consider lasers to maintain and build your collagen if you are over forty.
- Get a dermatologist's treatment and opinion if you have active acne during the perimenopausal time or during menopause.
- If wrinkles are surfacing and they bother you, start the repair process sooner rather than later.
- While estrogen replacement probably does help the skin a little, it has many other risks that can be serious.

PART SIX
FOCUS ON THE FUTURE

15

AN EFFECTIVE MAINTENANCE SCHEDULE—HERE'S HOW AND WHY

I've been trying for weeks to write about maintenance, but it hasn't been easy, and for a simple reason: maintenance takes up so much of my life that I barely have time to sit down at the computer.

—Nora Ephron

So, you've used some of your free time and your hard-earned money to repair the sun damage you had from baking on the seashore with baby oil instead of sunscreen. Now what?

Do you just ignore your skin and go back to your old wild ways? Or can you maintain your good-looking skin without breaking the bank or scheduling a weekly visit to your dermatologist?

You've made some significant gains. Your wrinkles are better, your jawline is tighter, you've gotten rid of the brown spots and red blood vessels, the lines around your mouth look better, and your frown lines have relaxed. So, what kind of maintenance should you schedule and when?

DEVELOPING A GOOD MAINTENANCE PLAN

Problem: To maintain your gains and slowly improve even more
Best solution: Develop a maintenance yearly worksheet that will help you organize your new skin-health schedule

Maintenance is much easier than repair. It's like a house: it's a lot easier to keep a nice house maintained than it is to fix up one that is run down. To maintain your newly improved skin should require only your daily care with products and a few visits a year to your dermatologist. After you've done the repair work, though (which certainly takes more effort for that first six months or a year), then there's really no need to be at your dermatologist any more than two to four times a year depending on your goals and your age.

Examples of Maintenance Schedules

Here are some sample maintenance schedules of several of my patients just so you can get an idea for what yours might look like. Yours will be, of course, individual to you and will depend on your age and what your specific skin issues are. Plan ahead and schedule your appointments well ahead of time to make sure you can get in before that vacation or your holiday parties. Whatever your work and social schedule, you should be able to make sure that you have at least seven to ten days before an important social event, because it's always possible to get a bruise.

Sample Schedule 1.   This is for a woman who is thirty-six years old and who likes to run and bike outdoors most of the year. She had a little acne, mostly on her forehead and chin, some early frown lines, and brown spots

February	Small amount of Botox in frown lines to relax them. A microdermabrasion or light peel to unclog pores, improve acne, and get skin glowing.
May	A presummer microdermabrasion or peel for acne—extra sunscreen if outdoors now
October	Yearly photorejuvenation treatment to remove any brown spots/freckles that have appeared after the summer. Botox treatment to relax frown lines. Maybe another microdermabrasion if acne still a problem.

and sun damage on her face. She's done with the repair phase now. She's on several prescription acne creams. Here's what she uses to maintain.

Sample Schedule 2.   This is for a woman who is forty-five years old and who spends a lot of time on her family sailboat in the summer and has moderate sun damage. She had some frown lines and lines from her nose to her mouth that were getting a little deeper. She has mild sagging at the jawline. She's done the repair—here's the maintenance.

February	These can both be scheduled in the same appointment: Botox for frown lines and one syringe of Juvederm to soften the lines from the nose to the mouth and the mouth to the chin.
June	Thermage full face (every other year) to prevent sagging along with Botox for frown lines. Possibly a syringe of Juvederm to soften lines from nose to mouth.
October	Yearly Fraxel treatment to remove any brown spots/freckles and improve wrinkles. Botox and Juvederm after the laser treatment to soften frown lines and lines from the nose to the mouth.

Sample Schedule 3.   This is the schedule for a sixty-eight-year-old woman whose skin texture was pretty good but who had some hollowing

November pre-holidays	Botox for frown lines, crow's feet, forehead lines, and lower face to relax upper lip lines; one to two syringes of Juvederm to maintain the lines from the nose to the chin, mouth to chin and "rehydrate" the lips. One syringe of CosmoPlast to fill in upper lip lines and define the lip border without adding volume.
February	Yearly Sculptra maintenance to prevent more sagging and fill hollows. Botox if needed.

May	Yearly laser photorejuvenation treatment to get rid of any brown spots or red broken blood vessels; possible fractional resurfacing if texture and wrinkles are more the problem. Botox full-face treatment. One to two syringes of Juvederm and one syringe of CosmoPlast like November.
August	Thermage yearly full-face and neck treatment to tighten the skin and prevent needing another facelift; touchup Botox and Juvederm, if needed.

and laxity with wrinkles through the cheek area. She has a very active social schedule and is involved in a lot of civic activities. She also has eight grandchildren and is tightly scheduled most of the time. She's done the repair—here's the maintenance.

Sample Schedule 4.   This patient is a fifty-four-year-old female with rosacea currently going through menopause (flushing). She tended to be red even prior to menopause. Other than the redness, she had some crow's feet and lines around the mouth. Uses sunscreen daily. She's done the repair—here's the maintenance.

October	Laser to reduce redness, either pulse-dye laser or photorejuvenation. Botox to the crow's feet area only (her forehead is fine). One syringe of Juvederm to fill in lines from the nose and mouth.
February	Second yearly laser to treat the redness, either pulse-dye laser or photorejuvenation. Thermage (yearly or every other year) to tighten skin and possibly to prevent needing a facelift.
June	Botox in crow's feet area only and one syringe of Juvederm.

THE BOTTOM LINE

The following overview will give you some idea of the time frames for general maintenance for different kinds of cosmetic treatments. Use this as a reference only, and be sure to develop your own plan in consultation with your dermatologist. You'll also find more personalized information on maintenance via the interactive profile at *www.yourskinplan.com*

- **Microdermabrasion:** You'll need an initial series of four or five, maintenance every four to six weeks for oily skin and as frequently as once every two weeks.
- **Botox:** For the first year, you may need injections every three to four months. After that, some patients need them only every five to six months.
- **Restylane or Juvederm:** You'll usually need injections every four to six months, or every six to nine months for the thicker forms Perlane and Juvederm Ultra Plus.
- **Sculptra:** After the first series of three or four treatments, you'll need maintenance of approximately one treatment each year.
- **Lasers for blood vessels and brown spots:** After the initial series of three to five treatments, you'll need one to two maintenance treatments per year, more if you spend a lot of time in the sun or flush a lot.
- **Laser hair removal:** After the initial series (usually four to eight treatments), you'll need maintenance at least once or twice per year, maybe more if you have hormone changes.
- **Thermage:** You'll need maintenance every two years and if you're over fifty, perhaps yearly.

16

FINDING A GOOD COSMETIC DERMATOLOGIST AND LASER CENTER

First, do no harm.

—*Hippocrates*

This is probably the most important chapter in the book. Regardless of what treatments you want done, if they're not done well, then you'll have wasted those two important things: your time and money, not to mention the risks of procedures gone wrong, which include infections and scarring, among others.

The difference between a great doctor (and laser center) and a just-okay one is that a great doctor will get consistently good results a higher percentage of the time. And, if you have a problem or complication, a great doctor will know how to fix the problem, and stand by his or her work and make sure that you get a good value for your money.

A not-so-great doctor will have more complications, not know how to fix the complications when they occur, and possibly not be fair with you about the money you've spent on something that didn't go well.

SEVEN QUESTIONS TO ASK ABOUT THE LASER CENTER YOU'RE CONSIDERING

1. *Is there a doctor on site?* This is regulated state by state and, believe it or not, some states do not require the medical director (that is,

237

the doctor) of a laser center to be on the premises any more than an hour or two a month. The doctor is the doctor *in name only* at these clinics. There is almost *no* physician training, supervision, or quality control for "technicians" to ensure that the lasers are set properly for the patients, that lasers are maintained properly, that treatments are done correctly, and that problems are handled promptly and well. Some states allow a laser trained PA-C or nurse practitioner to supervise laser use.

Ask: *"Is the doctor on site while the lasers are in operation, and will the doctor see me either at my consultation or at my first visit for actual laser treatment?"*

2. **Is the doctor board certified in dermatology?**   It's shocking, but there is no law preventing doctors from calling themselves whatever they want. Many centers all over the country are being set up by doctors who have absolutely no medical training in skin but who have decided that they want to cash in on skin services. Do you really want an anesthesiologist or gynecologist working on your face just because they've decided their lifestyle and income might be better if they inject Botox and buy some lasers? Yes, a pediatrician or a family-practice doctor can hang out their shingle and imply or directly state that they are a dermatologist. And there's no one to stop them from doing that!

The best way to find out if a doctor is board certified in dermatology is to go to the website AAD.org. This is the website for the American Academy of Dermatology, and it lists all the board-certified dermatologists.

Plastic surgeons are trained primarily to operate and have generally very little training in skin care other than wound management. In Seattle and other parts of the country, many plastic surgeons have added laser and injectable services but do not do those procedures themselves. Their main focus is surgery, so they hire nurses to do Botox and Restylane and lasers for them. My question is, how can they supervise someone doing a procedure when they may not be good at it themselves? It seems to me the doctor needs to know how to do the procedures in order to "supervise."

Ask: *"Who does the procedure, and how were they trained?"*

3. **Have they been in business for more than five years?**   This is also a key question, because many "skin clinics" and mini-spas fail within the first three to five years. They may start well initially, with heavy advertising to bring in customers. But they often cannot sustain a high level of results and safety over a broad spectrum of their customer base. So they go out of business, leaving in their wake a trail of lawsuits, unhappy and sometimes scarred patients, and patients who have paid money for services that they never received.

If the doctor and laser center have been in business more than five years and are well known in the community, chances are they're operating to a higher standard of medicine and are treating their patients fairly. Prices are often surprisingly comparable, so the question is, Whom do you trust with your face?

Ask: *"How long have you been in business in this location?"*

4. **Do they advertise?**   Doctors who are good and have been in business for a while are busy. It's expensive to advertise. The only reason for a doctor to advertise is if they don't have enough patients. If the doctor doesn't have enough patients, the question is, Why not? Frequently the answer is not something you really want to know. Great doctors usually don't advertise because they have all the patients they need. Their referrals come from their patients and other doctors. Or they may have been seen on TV or radio as an expert (a paid advertisement doesn't count). If you hear or see a lot of print advertisement, radio or TV advertising, be concerned.

Ask: *"Do you advertise on TV, radio, or print?"*

5. **Who does the lasering?**   I think it is very reasonable for a board-certified dermatologist or plastic surgeon who is laser and injectable trained and experienced themselves to delegate lasers or injectables to registered RNs, ARNPs, or PA-C, or some MAs (all medical providers) who are directly trained and supervised by that doctor. Medical providers have the medical training, experience, and judgment to operate lasers and handle complications in conjunction with a physician, with the goal of giving their patients excellent-quality laser treatments in a safe environment.

All too often in shady clinics the lasering is being done by a "tech," who is an individual with absolutely no medical education whatsoever and who is operating with little or no training in an unsupervised environment.

Again, **ask:** *"Does the person doing the lasering or injectable on me have any medical education? What is their degree or certificate?"*

6.   ***Don't buy or commit to anything at the consult.***   Cosmetic procedures are luxuries. No one is dying, and no immediate surgery is needed. Good laser centers that operate ethically will never try to "hard sell" you or get you to commit your money before you walk out the door. An excellent center *wants* you to think over what's involved, read all the materials they've given you, and have some time to decide if that's really what you want to do. Don't be fooled by slick salespeople or bargains that are offered if you book today rather than later. Think before you commit to services or buy a lot of products at your first visit to an office.

Ask yourself: *"Do I feel pressured to buy products or to book treatments at my first visit?"*

7.   ***Don't be persuaded by before-and-after photographs.***   Deeply ingrained in us is the idea that seeing is believing. In this day of modern photography, we need to be suspicious of photos. There are two problems with before and after photographs.

The first problem is that companies and doctors will always put their absolutely best before and after photographs on a website or post them in their office. When you look at that photo, you don't know whether one out of one hundred people who had the procedure got that kind of result or whether ninety-five out of one hundred people who had that procedure got that result. It's very easy to hit a home run with the occasional patient. What matters, though, is getting consistently great results over a wide spectrum of patients. You just don't know if that photograph is representative or not.

The second problem is that with current ability to alter digital images, you really can't know whether that photograph is accurate or represents something that has been altered.

Ask: *"Am I likely to get a result that is like the one I'm seeing in the photograph?"* That answer is only as good as the honesty and ethics of the office.

WHAT TO ASK YOUR FRIENDS

Friends can be a good, but not perfect, source of information. Remember to consider the source. Some of your friends may be accurate sources of information. Others may be positive about almost everything (uncritical) or critical of almost everything (never happy). Use your friends as resources but don't consider them the final word.

Ask specifically what your friend liked about the doctor and the office. More specific information is more helpful than the more general. Ask: "Was the doctor's staff helpful and friendly?" "Was it easy to get all the information about whatever you were having done?" "Did you have enough time with the doctor and the staff?" "Did the doctor run pretty much on time?" If your friend had questions later on, were they answered promptly and courteously by phone? This just gives you an idea. There may be other things that are important to you.

Look at your friend's face! One of the best recommendations for a cosmetic dermatologist is how their patients look. Is your friend's skin gradually getting better and better? Does her skin quality and appearance seem to be improving slowly while yours is not? Does her skin have a healthy glow? Are injectables like Botox and Restylane used with a light and gentle hand (rather than giving the frozen or overstuffed look). The answer to your question, "Is the doctor good?" may be right in front of your eyes.

HOW TO HAVE A GOOD RELATIONSHIP WITH YOUR DOCTOR

Once you've found a good doctor, it's nice to have a good relationship with her or him. Doctors are human, after all, and they appreciate patients who respect their time and experience.

Here are things you can do to make it go well. It goes without saying that a good doctor should run on time (or within fifteen to thirty minutes max), be focused on you when you're there, be open to a reasonable number of questions, explain things clearly and provide excellent nursing support for further education and call backs.

Here's what you can do to avoid being a "nightmare" patient. These are the patients who

- **Don't read the written literature and consent forms given them.** And then come to the next appointment wanting the doctor and staff to spend twenty minutes answering all the questions that were covered in the written materials.
- **Want everything to improve instantly.** Even after it's been explained over and over that improvement is gradual and that a series of treatments (not just one) will give the best results.
- **Are "Web" experts.** Some people get information online, think everything they read online is true, and expect their doctors to spend a lot of time explaining to them why the misinformation they read on the web is faulty, incomplete, not pertinent to their situation, or just plain marketing hype.
- **Are late, rude to staff members, and don't show up or cancel frequently.** Office staff are like everyone else in that you will get better care and favors done if you are on time, considerate, and start from the assumption that everyone *is* really trying to help you. Busy doctors often have other patients who would like to be seen. If you really must cancel, it's nice to explain the reason.
- **Have no sense of boundaries.** These patients consistently add more things that they want the doctor to address, usually at the end of a visit. They call back three to four times after every visit and constantly want extra favors. For example, it's fine to ask that the doctor come by for a quick check on your laser progress when you're in for a laser treatment with the nurse. But it isn't appropri-

ate to ask that doctor to do an entire evaluation of your chronic and difficult acne at the same time. Schedule a separate appointment for the separate problem of acne.

WHAT TO ASK ABOUT YOUR DOCTOR

Is your dermatologist really a dermatologist? Believe it or not, once a doctor graduates from medical school and does an internship, she or he can legally call herself anything she wants. A family practitioner or somebody board-certified in urology can decide he wants to call himself a dermatologist. In my opinion, this is unethical, but unfortunately it is legal. To make sure that your dermatologist is for real, double check that he or she has board certification in dermatology (go to *www.aad.org*).

Physician residency programs.   Most patients have a really difficult time evaluating a doctor's credentials. For instance, you probably won't really know which residency programs are outstanding ones, whether the doctor graduated with honors in medical school, or whether he was at the top of his residency program. Some dermatologists have websites where they post their credentials. Look for honors such as Alpha Omega Alpha (which is the honor society in medical school), and look for any national awards or grants. As far as residency programs go, you can't assume that a state university residency program is less prestigious than a private university program, like Harvard. Some large state universities' dermatology training programs are ranked higher than some of the Ivy League residency training programs.

University affiliation.   You might think this would be meaningful, but it often isn't. Many doctors will list what is called a "clinical faculty appointment" (such as associate clinical professor). This is a title given to doctors in private practice who volunteer a small amount of time each year to teach residents. Often, it amounts to a half day a week for a month or two a year. This type of clinical faculty appointment is not the same as being a professor. The term *clinical professor* is often used to designate doctors who are in private practice but who help at the university periodically.

Laser education.   Laser education is even more difficult to evaluate because many dermatologists who trained in the 1980s or 1990s came from residency programs where training in cosmetic dermatology didn't exist because the field was new. This has gradually been changing over the past ten years, and now in this decade some of the dermatology residents coming out of training have fairly extensive training in cosmetic and laser dermatology. Older doctors had to actively seek laser and cosmetic training courses, preceptorships, and workshops. Again, the reputation of the doctor and the length of time that she has been in practice are going to be more important than where she graduated from.

WHOM TO AVOID

This is a tough one because there are many different types of excellent doctors out there. You may not click with a particular one even though his work is excellent. Since there are many excellent cosmetic dermatologists in practice now (see the regional guide in the Resources section at the back), it's important to understand there is a wide range of patient styles and doctor styles. Sometimes it's just a matter of making a good fit. But here are some good general guidelines:

Avoid medi-spas.   unless the doctor is onsite full-time and is board-certified in dermatology or plastic surgery. If the onsite doctor is board-certified in a specialty like anesthesiology, orthopedics, urology, or ob-gyn, it means he or she has had little or no training in skin. These doctors do not know how to deal with complications (I know because I have seen many of their complications in my own clinic).

Avoid laser centers that offer "specials."   While it is very reasonable to compare prices at two or three reputable centers, be suspicious if a center is significantly less expensive than others. This is an area, like plastic surgery, where shopping for bargain basement prices isn't a great idea. The best dermatologic laser surgeons will usually charge somewhere from the median to the higher end of the cost spectrum because they are better and are usually busy. They also often have a greater variety of laser equipment, which increases their costs. Also, excellent laser physicians tend to have excellent staff that they treat respectfully and pay well. Laser costs vary by geographical area.

Use your eyes.   High quality comes from the top down. When you go in for your consultation look around you. Is the office clean and aesthetically pleasing? Is the staff professionally dressed, helpful, and caring? Are forms kept to a minimum and patient friendly? Is the nursing staff positive, energetic, and eager to help you? Are there patient-education materials to take home and read when time permits? And lastly, are your follow-up questions answered promptly and courteously?

SCHEDULING YOUR FIRST APPOINTMENT

Many people feel uncomfortable calling a doctor's office and are uncertain about what exactly they want. Before you make that call, read the following so you know a bit better what you want. You'll save yourself and the doctor's office time and confusion.

Do you want a cosmetic consultation or a medical appointment? Many dermatologists do both medical and cosmetic dermatology. I know that we have occasionally had patients who scheduled for the wrong thing. If you need a medical appointment, then it's easy. Just say you need an appointment for your acne, rosacea, mole check, etc. Once you are there for your medical appointment, it's okay to ask the doctor for some preliminary information about cosmetic treatments.

Please remember though, that you scheduled a medical appointment, and your doctor probably won't be able to spend a lot of time with you on a cosmetic matter. I will often do a very brief evaluation and give my medical patients some information and an appointment for a cosmetic visit or consultation in the future.

If you schedule a cosmetic consultation, then it helps to know what you are interested in. For example, you might be interested in Botox treatments or a filler, lasers to repair sun damage or wrinkles. It's okay to be unsure about this, but it is helpful for the staff to know if you are more interested in injectables (like Botox) or more interested in lasers or both. There may be a charge for a cosmetic consultation ranging anywhere from $50 to $250 depending on the doctor and the city.

Very often, initial consultations will be with one of the nursing or consultation staff. The nurse will meet with you, do a preliminary assessment, give you information, and help you prioritize what you'd like to fix. Often the doctor is available at the end of the consultation to answer further questions and help with deciding exactly what technology to use. If you want to make sure that you will see the doctor at the consultation, be sure you tell the front office coordinator or receptionist when you book your appointment, in case the doctor is traveling.

Bring a list to your first appointment. Prepare a list of your concerns. This will help the cosmetic nurse specialist and your dermatologist answer most of your questions. Your conversation is really an opportunity to get to know the doctor and his/her staff and understand all of the options available to treat you. You should never be given the "hard sell" at a consultation. Be wary of centers where you are offered a discount to schedule on the same day. It's fine to book your appointment that day if *you* want to, but resist offices that are pressuring you heavily to do so before you leave the office.

YOUR COSMETIC CONSULTATION

Look for a warm, individual approach to this, not a cookie-cutter format. The nurse and doctor should not only give you basic information, but they should also answer any questions and concerns that you may have. The consultation should cover the following:

- information about how this particular treatment will help you achieve your goals
- a detailed account of how the treatment is done and approximately how many treatments will be needed

- any preparations you need to do prior to the treatment
- what to expect during the treatment (including any possible complications)
- what type of care you'll need after the procedure and if there are any restrictions on your activities
- a brief review of your skin-care program to make sure it includes a good quality sunscreen and state-of-the-art products to help reverse sun damage
- the expected cost of the procedure

After the consultation, the nurse will often send you a letter summarizing your discussion. You should be given his or her phone number, so that if you have questions after you've reviewed the written material you can call someone with in-depth knowledge.

PA-CS, ARNPS, AND RNS IN A DOCTOR'S PRACTICE

There is a lot of confusion in the general public about medical certifications and what they actually mean. PA-Cs and ARNPs are often referred to as "physician extenders" or "midlevel providers." Such practitioners have not gone to medical school but have the training and authority to diagnose and treat problems of a limited nature and have limited authority to write prescriptions.

PA-Cs.   This stands for *physician's assistant certified.* A newer midlevel provider role, it's a certification area that is growing rapidly. PAs have four years of college and then an intensive two-year training program that includes some practical education. Many PAs also have many years of practice in a health-care field, such as being an emergency medical technician in the fire department, an RN, a medic in the military, or having a background in pharmaceutical sales.

A doctor, by comparison, has four years of college, four years of medical school, and between three and six years of specialized residency training. For example, I had four years of college, four years of medical school, three years of internal medicine residency and three years of dermatology residency training. Then I stayed on the full-time faculty for a year at a university before going into private practice.

The length, depth, and breadth of knowledge in a doctor's training are vastly greater than a PA's or ARNP's. This is why PA-Cs and ARNPs usually must practice under the supervision of a doctor, though it varies by state how close that supervision has to be. Ideally, the physician and the PA-C would practice onsite together rather than the PA-C (other than in very rural areas) being at another site. PA-Cs can provide excellent care in a supervised setting.

ARNPs.   This stands for a *registered nurse practitioner.* These are nurses (RNs) who have undergone extra specialty training in areas like family medicine, gynecology, pediatrics, or dermatology. They have often had many years of prior experience in their particular areas and often have gone back to school for one or two years to increase their certification from RN to ARNP. Again, they are midlevel providers with limited prescribing authority. They can also be an excellent source of care. In some states, they are allowed to practice medicine without direct physician supervision.

LPNs and MAs.   Other personnel working in a physician's office may include LPNs (*licensed practical nurses*). They generally have gone to a two-year community college nursing program as opposed to a four-year, more rigorous private or public university program that is required to get an RN. MA stands for *medical assistant.* MAs generally have had one year of medical assistance training and are not required to have a college degree in order to get an MA. LPNs are also not required to have a college degree.

Laser "Technicians." A laser technician does not have any kind of medical education, degree, or license. This "technician" category (in my opinion) was invented to make people with no medical background or education sound legitimate to operate a medical device like a laser. Often, the only training that many of these "laser techs" have had is a one-or two-day training seminar given by the laser company.

Many states now are regulating who, in fact, can use a laser and what constitutes laser supervision. In my opinion, a laser technician with no medical education or licensing should never be operating a laser. If the laser center tells you that a technician will be treating you, ask them exactly what that means and what medical education that person has had.

THE BOTTOM LINE

- Ask the seven questions when considering a laser center.
- Ask your friends who they see and what they like, but don't take it as gospel.
- Come prepared to your appointment or consultation.
- Don't let yourself be pressured into committing to cosmetic procedures. There's no rush!
- Try to be a great patient once you've found a good doctor, to keep your relationship positive.

17

NEW AND EMERGING TECHNOLOGIES

For a successful technology, reality must take precedence over public relations, for Nature cannot be fooled.
—*Richard Feynman*

In this chapter, I'll give you an update on the most frequently asked-about technologies, together with my unvarnished opinion of them. (I own many lasers and a "blu" light device in my own clinic, but I pay for all my lasers and have no financial ties of any kind to any of the companies who make any of these devices or technologies). Some technologies are in this chapter because, although they are not new in the past year or two, the uses for them are still evolving rapidly. As these technologies are used by more doctors and patients, we will get more data on their results, risks and complications.

You would think this would all be worked out before a new laser or device is marketed to the public and sold to doctors. Not so. If anything, technology is being released earlier as companies try to get a competitive advantage in the marketplace.

Here are the "newer" technologies I'll cover:

- fractional laser resurfacing
- photodynamic or "blu light" therapy
- mesotherapy

- nanosphere technology
- LED–light-emitting diode devices

FRACTIONAL LASER RESURFACING

Some doctors will object to this being put in new technology but there are two good reasons for it to be mentioned here. First, some of the best uses and exact settings for the Fraxel, the oldest of the fractional lasers, have been worked out but many have not. There is a lot of evolving research and clinical experience with this laser. Second, there are now at least six competing lasers in the fractional category. These are divided further into ablative (visibly removes a layer of skin) and nonablative (does this more microscopically). There are a lot of unanswered questions about how and if these compare to the Fraxel.

What Is It?

Traditional laser resurfacing used a carbon dioxide laser to do a controlled burn of the skin. Then new skin would regrow. Results for wrinkles were usually excellent. But carbon dioxide resurfacing and deeper erbium-laser resurfacing left raw skin and required twoweeks immediate healing followed sometimes by months of redness and sun sensitivity.

Then someone had the bright idea of taking that laser beam and breaking it into thousands of small beams (the laser beam is cut up or "fractionated"). These tiny, pixilated beams cause far less injury to the skin, primarily because the fractionated beams leave areas of undamaged skin around all the little pixilated beams of laser light. So the healing time is far less. Each treatment with a Fraxel laser replaces about 15 to 20 percent of your skin.

It is true that patients need three or four treatments with the fractional laser, but they can walk out of each treatment with only some redness and without the raw skin caused by the older resurfacing technology. Also, since the entire top layer of skin is not being taken off, there are far fewer risks of infection and scarring.

Why Is this Technology Emerging?

The fractional technology is relatively new with a lot of promise, but we are only at the beginning of the learning curve. There are currently five fractional resurfacing lasers on the market, and I am sure there will be several more in the next few years.

For the techies among you, the best-known fractional lasers are the Fraxel (a fractionated 1,550 nanometer fiber laser), the ActiveFX (a fractionated carbon dioxide laser), the Affirm (a fractionated 1440 nanometer Nd:YAG laser), the Lux 1540 (a fractionated 1540 nanometer Er:Yag laser), and the Harmony (a fractionated 2,940 nanometer Er:YAG laser). You get the picture: there's a lot going on.

The two big questions are which of these devices will prove over the long term to be the most useful and able to live up to its marketing claims (no small feat); and two, what are the best ways to use these lasers in terms of which skin sites are improved the most by them, which problems respond the best, how many treatments are needed, and at what energy levels? These are all still under discussion in the laser community.

These questions have not been answered definitively. This is in contrast, for example, to hair-removal technology or technology for photorejuvenation with IPLs, where the optimal use for patients' problems and exact parameters for the lasers have been largely worked out over the last five to ten years.

This is where the much-needed research that I mentioned above is so important. We still don't know which of these devices will turn out to be the best over the long term. Fraxel was the first of these fractionated lasers to come to market and has had the most press. That doesn't necessarily mean that it's the best of these technologies. Only time and research will determine which one of these, if any, is a clear leader in terms of results, or if, in fact, they are all nearly equivalent.

My Vote

If you live near a center that has been using Fraxels or one of the other fractional laser devices for several years, and it is run ethically, and they get consistently good results, then I would recommend going ahead. Otherwise, I think it is best to wait, particularly if your budget is tight and you can't afford to spend three thousand to five thousand dollars to get perhaps a less-than-great result. Time will definitely sort out which of these devices is best and under what circumstances they work best.

PHOTODYNAMIC OR "BLU LIGHT" THERAPY

What Is It?

Photodynamic or "Blu Light" therapy involves painting a clear liquid (aminolevulinic acid or ALA) on the skin and then incubating it for thirty minutes to two hours (sometimes longer than that). You can read or do other things while you wait as long as you have no sun exposure.

The ALA is a compound found inside of our red blood cells. It is completely natural and is produced in the laboratory. What the ALA does is make your skin, and precancerous lesions on the skin, very sensitive to certain wavelengths of light. The light, whether it's a laser source or a pure blue light, for example, causes activation of the ALA which then selectively damages cells to achieve a purpose. This process, originally developed for precancerous spots, has now gone on to be used for other problems, including acne and sun-damaged skin.

Why Is It Emerging?

There is a certain unpredictability when a laser or a blue or red light is combined with ALA. The incubation time for the ALA and the light source to activate is still under discussion. A recent study showed that even ambient light (normal room light) activates it somewhat.

Having said that, in an experienced center that does this therapy correctly, a very nice result can be obtained, as long as you are willing to accept the fact that you may have some visible redness and peeling—in other words, downtime—for several days or up to a week or so.

I have seen patients from other offices where the patient was told that this would be a no-downtime procedure. The patients were *not* happy to find that, in fact, they could not go to work for a number of days due to redness and peeling. In my office, we use photodynamic therapy (ALA with blu light or IPL laser) for precancerous lesions. We generally don't use it for sun damage or acne because my patients don't want the unpredictability or any downtime.

Sun-damaged skin. For sun-damaged skin and cosmetic reasons, the ALA has been most often combined with an intense pulse light laser (IPL). The ALA solution again is painted on the skin, incubated for a period of usually thirty to sixty minutes, and then activated with the laser light. Expert centers only please.

I recently saw a patient with a terrible burn from another office where a peel had been done, then the ALA had been painted on, and then the ALA was activated with the laser. The woman had second-degree burns over her entire chest and has had, as you can imagine, some problems healing. This therapy for cosmetic purposes should not be undertaken lightly. It can go, and sometimes does go, terribly wrong.

Some doctors argue that they can get the same result with two or three ALA plus laser as with a series of five IPL treatments. If you don't mind risking an unpredictable result that might take you out of your social activities or work for several days unexpectedly, then go ahead. The cost of the two series is about the same because the cost per treatment of ALA with IPL is greater than the cost per treatment of the IPL alone.

We use aggressive IPL without the ALA for the simple reason my patients don't want any downtime. We get excellent, predictable, no-downtime results with a series of five IPL treatments.

Acne. Light therapy with ALA is also used for acne. The ALA does seem to soak in, at least some, to the oil glands. When the light activates the ALA, it causes redness and often peeling, which improves acne over a series of treatments. Sometimes there is a little peeling, sometimes a lot.

This is also not a cure-all for acne. In fact, there is no cure-all for acne, except perhaps Accutane for cystic acne. But Accutane is a prescription drug that must be carefully monitored. Light therapy with ALA can be part of a whole regimen aimed at good acne control.

Dermatologists will also use prescription antiacne creams or gels, oral contraceptives, oral antibiotics, lasers, or perhaps microdermabrasion or other light peels when a patient has a lot of plugged pores. Again, there is no one cure-all for acne, only different strategies that work for different patients.

My Vote

I vote no to ALA plus IPL for cosmetic reasons, because there is too much redness and peeling with downtime, and there is really not much cost savings.

I vote yes for treatment of acne if many other treatments have failed and for treatment of precancerous lesions (usually paid for by medical insurance) to ALA plus blue light.

MESOTHERAPY

What Is It?

Mesotherapy is a system of injecting a mixture of vitamins, minerals, enzymes, and other chemicals into the skin with the intent of changing body contours or improving skin quality.

Why Is This Technology Emerging?

Mesotherapy has been used for many years in Europe, particularly in France. It is important to note that there have been no controlled studies of mesotherapy to date. So, this means that all the information about mesotherapy is now gotten from the people who are doing the mesotherapy and, as you can imagine, they have a significant financial stake in mesotherapy treatments. Therefore, my conclusion is that pretty much everything that is said about mesotherapy needs to be taken with a large grain of salt. There are many unanswered questions.

Safety

My concern is that the safety of mesotherapy has not been fully evaluated. While there have been no deaths reported (to my knowledge), there have been reports of complications, such as rashes that produced lumps and bumps in the skin and depressions in the skin that could not be corrected. Some of these complications were permanent and on the face.

Unanswered questions include what are the drugs used in mesotherapy (many of the solutions don't list what's in them), and how much of the drugs in the mesotherapy cocktails are being absorbed into the body through the bloodstream and at what levels. Some of the ingredients in the mesotherapy cocktails are soluble in fat cells, which may mean that there is long-term storage of the drug with possible consequences later. What is each ingredient doing both alone and in combination? Some mesotherapy solutions have been found to contain more than twenty different ingredients, with little being known about which of those ingredients might be effective, what happens when you mix them, and which might be toxic.

When you go for a mesotherapy injection, you may have no idea what is being put into the solutions since there is no standardization or FDA review of these solutions. For example, one mesotherapy ingredient is something called isoproterenol, which is an FDA-approved pharmaceutical. Isoproterenol is an antiarrhythmic (heart) medication and is part of the sequence used by medics to revive someone's heart after he or she has died. It is being used in mesotherapy solutions with little idea of what the safety implications are for the injection of this drug into the skin. This is just one example of the many ingredients used in mesotherapy solutions.

My Vote

No. Stay away from these until there is some general agreement and standardization of what actually belongs in the mesotherapy solution and at what concentration. We need to have more knowledge about what complications might occur and how to prevent them.

NANOSPHERE TECHNOLOGY

What Is It?

You are probably thinking, "Why should I care about nanotechnology?" You'll be seeing this term used more and more on all sorts of cosmetics from makeup to antiaging skin creams. Nanotechnology is a catch-all phrase for materials and devices that operate at the nano scale. Nano is just a unit of measurement. For example, a nanometer is one billionth of a meter.

To give you an idea, a human red blood cell is over two thousand nanometers long, which is pretty much outside the nano-scale range. Nanotechnology is being used in dozens of different industries, including such diverse areas as commercial electric motors, flat-screen television displays, sensing devices, aerospace, pharmaceuticals, and the cosmetics industry.

Uses in skin.   Nanosphere technology was first used, and has been used for at least a decade now, in certain types of sunscreens containing zinc. The zinc is used for its ultraviolet radiation absorbing properties but can be white. The nanoparticles' small size makes them invisible to the eye, and so the lotion is clear rather than white. When it comes to zinc, a mineral found in our own bodies, and thought, at least in reasonable amounts, to be healthy, there really isn't too much of a problem.

The problem is that nanoparticles are now being used in all types of cosmetics. Because they are cosmetics, they do not have to be reviewed by the FDA and, unless something goes wrong (which could be way in the future), there is little or no regulation of the product.

The problem is we don't know where these tiny little particles, which can make their way through the skin, go after they are in the body. Do they then land in the delicate tissues of the lung only to possibly cause lung problems later? Could they be transmitted to the brain where an accumulation of a certain nano-sized chemicals might have long-term implications for brain function? We just don't know at this point.

Unlike pharmaceuticals, cosmetics don't have to pass a safety test before they are sold to the public. Just because zinc and titanium nanoparticles have been used in sunscreens for ten to fifteen years doesn't mean that other chemicals are equally safe.

My Vote

Yes, for sunscreens because nanoparticles have been used now for ten to fifteen years with no reported ill effects, and zinc is natural in our bodies. A strong caution on all the rest of the cosmeceuticals.

LIGHT-EMITTING DIODES (LEDS)

What Is It?

These devices emit low levels of certain wavelengths of light to try to trigger natural intracellular repair processes.

Why Is It Emerging?

The goal of these treatments (usually done in a series and then with regular maintenance) is to stimulate your skin to retain its collagen, reduce inflammation and other possible benefits. The one group of patients who has been shown to clearly benefit is those undergoing radiation for breast cancer. The LED treatments reduced inflammation and caused fewer skin reactions potentially disrupting therapy.

The key is all the unanswered questions. Some of the LED's effects are known, but what might be other, longer term effects that aren't known? The results tend to be subtle. Are the results really worth the extra expense and time it takes? Are there any bad effects? Many of the studies haven't been controlled well. It seems to work for acne, at least somewhat, but does it work any better than the many tried and true treatments we already have?

My Vote

Wait on this one until there's more research and clinical experience.

THE BOTTOM LINE

- yes on fractional resurfacing (like Fraxel) if you live near an experienced laser center in a metropolitan area and money is not tight.
- yes for precancerous lesions with ALA and blue light, but no on photodynamic treatments with ALA with lasers for cosmetic purposes
- no on mesotherapy
- yes on nanosphere techonology for mineral (zinc) sunscreens, but no for now on other cosmeceuticals
- no for now on light-emitting diode devices until better, larger studies are done

18

KNOWLEDGE IS POWER

My goal in this book has been to give you power. Power to think about products and select them without being manipulated by the persuasive ad campaigns of big companies. Power to learn about your own face and what to expect from modern cosmetic dermatology in terms of enhancing it. Power to find and work with a good doctor. Power to spend your money wisely.

All of this is important now more than ever before as cosmetic services are springing up in sports clubs, salons, and "medi-spas." As this trend accelerates, the line between medical expertise and the profit motive in cosmetic services is becoming more and more blurred. How do you know, for instance, if the technician performing your laser treatment is experienced and effective, or if he just got trained the day before by a laser company representative? How do you know if the new treatment being promoted is effective and safe? Or that the product line offered is any good?

You need the information to give you the power to find the best treatments and care. If you've spent some time with this book, I know that you're already better armed to make good decisions about your own skin care and antiaging efforts.

Sometimes patients are surprised when I ask them what their goal is with a certain issue. "I want to fix this," they say. Or, "I want to look younger, of course." And I agree, we all want to repair some of the damage we've done with sun exposure, too much of whatever, and just plain aging. We all want to look a little younger.

But most of my patients don't want to look artificial. They don't want to look as if they've had a lot of surgery. They may want to appear five or ten years younger, but they still want to look like themselves just refreshed and rested, as I like to say.

And that is a wonderful goal. Some of my happiest days are when I see a patient look at herself in the mirror after a treatment and she sees the improvement in her skin or on her face. She stands just a bit straighter; she looks more alive. That improvement in her skin and face translates into a small but very significant improvement in her overall confidence. And I'm a firm believer that confidence is contagious; when women and men are feeling confident, they feel better and treat others better. So, good luck as you undertake your surgery-free makeover—may it bring you much happiness, confidence, and restore your youthful glow!

RESOURCES*

STATE	CITY		CONTACT INFORMATION
Arizona	Phoenix	Dermatologist	Romine, Kristine MD Camelback Dermatology and Skin Surgery 4350 E. Camelback Rd. #A200 Phoenix, AZ 85018 Phone: (602) 954-7546 Fax: (602) 952-294 www.camelbackderm.com
Arizona	Scottsdale	Dermatologist	Linder, Jennifer MD 8501 N. Scottsdale Road Scottsdale, AZ 85253 Phone: (480) 946-7939 www.jenniferlindermd.com
Arizona	Scottsdale	Dermatologist	McCraken, Gary MD 14275 N. Eighty-seventh Street #110 Scottsdale, AZ 85260 Phone: (480) 905-8485 Fax: (480) 905-7274 www.northscottsdalederm.com
Arizona	Tucson	Dermatologist	Comstock, Jody MD 1845 W. Orange Grove Rd., #101 Tucson, AZ 85704 Phone: (520) 797-8885 www.skinspectrum.com
California	Campbell	Dermatologist	Noodleman, Richard MD 3803 S. Bascom Avenue Suite 200 Campbell, CA 95008-7317 Phone: (408) 559-0988 Fax: (408) 369-4263 www.agedefy.com

* There are many other excellent centers with board certified dermatologists.

California	Beverly Hills	Dermatologist	Schaffran, Robin MD 8920 Wilshire Boulevard #545 Beverly Hills, CA 90211 Phone: (310) 854-3003 Fax: (310) 854-0811
California	Del Mar	Dermatologist	Atkin, Deborah MD Dermatology and Laser Center of Delmar 12865 Pointe Del Mar Way Suite 160 Del Mar, CA 92014-3860 Phone: (858) 350-7546 Fax: (858) 350-8282 www.dermdelmar.com
California	Irvine	Dermatologist	Zachary, Christopher B. MD University of California, Irvine 22 Silhouette Irvine, CA 92603 Phone: (924) 824-5515 Fax: (924) 824-7454 czachary@uci.edu
California	La Jolla	Dermatologist	Butterwick, Kimberly J. MD 7630 Fay Avenue La Jolla, CA 92037 Phone: (858) 459-7011 www.spa-md.com
California	Los Altos		Green, Brad MD 3130 Alpine Road Los Altos, CA (650) 851-0155
California	Los Altos	Dermatologist	Berman, Dave MD 900 Welch Road Suite 300 Los Altos, CA 94304 Phone: (650) 325-6000 Fax: (650) 325-8091 www.bermanmd.com

California	Los Angeles	Dermatologist	Moy, Ronald MD Moy-Fincher Medical Group 100 UCLA Medical Plaza Suite 590 Los Angeles, CA 90024-6992 Phone: (310) 794-7422
California	Los Gatos	Dermatologist	Bitter, Patrick MD Advanced Aesthetic Dermatology 14651 S. Bascom Way Los Gatos 95032 Phone: (408) 358-5757 Fax: (408) 358-8951 www.fotofacial.com
California	Palo Alto	Dermatologist	Rahman, Zakia MD Stanford University 37171 Sycamore Street Suite 1027 Palo Alto, CA 94560 Phone: (650) 246-1785 Fax: (650) 605-2855 dermasurgerymd@gmail.com
California	Sacramento	Dermatologist	Kilmer, Suzanne MD Chotzen, Vera A. MD Laser & Skin Surgery Center of Northern California 3835 J Street Sacramento, CA 95816 Phone: (916) 456-0400 fax: (916) 456-0499
California	Sacramento	Dermatologist	Tanghetti, Emil A. MD Center for Dermatology & Laser Surgery 5601 J Street Sacramento, CA 95819 Phone: (916) 454-5922 Fax: (916) 454-2156 et@mgci.com

California	San Francisco	Dermatologist	Matarasso, Seth MD 490 Post Street Suite 700 San Francisco 94102 Phone: (415) 362-2238 Fax: (415) 362-7745
California	San Francisco	Dermatologist	Narukar, Victor A. MD Bay Area Laser Institute 2100 Webster Street Suite 505 San Francisco, CA 94115 phone: (415) 923-3377 fax: (415) 923-3277
California	San Diego	Dermatologist	Mauricio, Tess MD Scripps Ranch Dermatology Center 9999 Mira Mesa Boulevard Suite 103 San Diego, CA 92131 phone: (858) 689-4990 www.scrippsderm.com
California	San Diego	Dermatologist	Ross, E. Victor Jr. MD Scripps Clinic 3811 Valley Centre Drive San Diego, CA 92130 Phone: (858) 764-9042 Fax: (858) 764-9041 Ross.edward@scrippshealth.org
California	San Jose	Dermatologist	Colby, Sara L. MD 2400 Samaritan Drive Suites 103 & 203 San Jose, CA 95124 Phone: (408) 369-5600 www.slcskin.com
California	Santa Monica	Dermatologist	Grossman, Karen MD 1301 Twentieth Street Santa Monica, CA 90404 Phone: (310) 998-0040 www.grossmandermatology.com

California	Santa Monica	Dermatologist	Shamban, Ava T. MD Laser Institute and European Skin Care 2021 Santa Monica Boulevard, #600-E Santa Monica, CA 90404-2208 Phone: (310) 828-2282 Fax: (310) 828-8504
California	Torrance	Dermatologist	Duffy, David MD 4201 Torrance Boulevard Suite 710 Torrance, CA 90503-4510 Phone: (310) 370-5670 www.drdavidmduffy.com
Colorado	Englewood	Dermatologist	Cohen, Joel MD About Skin Dermatology 499 E. Hampden Avenue Suite 450 Englewood, CO 80113 Phone: (303) 756-SKIN (7546) Fax: (303) 756-7547 www.aboutskinderm.com
Connecticut	New Haven	Dermatologist	Donofrio, Lisa M. MD The Savin Center 134 Park Street New Haven, CT 06511-5409 Phone: (203) 865-6143 Fax: (203) 772-1265 www.savincenter.com
District of Columbia	Washington	Dermatologist	Alster, Tina S. MD Tanzi, Elizabeth L. MD Washington Institute of Dermatologic Laser Surgery 1430 K Street NW #200 Washington, DC 20005 Phone: (202) 628-8855 Fax: (202) 628-8850 www.skinlaser.com etanzi@skinlaser

Florida	Miami	Dermatologist	Baumann, Leslie MD 1295 NW Fourteenth Street Suite K Miami, FL 33125 Phone: (305) 324-7546 Fax: (305) 324-9249 www.skintypesolutions.com
Florida	Coral Gables	Dermatologist	Brandt, Fredric S. MD 4425 Ponce De Leon Blvd # 200 Coral Gables, FL 33146 Phone: (305) 443-6606 Fax: (305) 443-04890 www.drbrandtskincare.com
Florida	West Palm Beach	Dermatologist	Beer, Kenneth MD Palm Beach Esthetic Center 1500 North Dixie Highway Suite #305 West Palm Beach, FL 33401 Phone: (561) 655-9055 Fax: (561) 655-9233 www.palmbeachcosmetic.com
Georgia	Alpharetta	Dermatologist	Tiffani Hamilton, MD 4165 Old Milton Pkwy, Suite 150 Alpharetta, GA 30005 Phone: (770) 360-8881 www.dermandvein.com
Georgia	Atlanta	Dermatologist	Brody, Harold J. MD 1218 West Paces Ferry Road #200 Atlanta, GA 30327 Phone: (404) 525-7409
Idaho	Rigby	Dermatologist	Bishop, Kay MD 403 N. 4000 E. Rigby, ID 83442 Phone: (208) 745-0200 Fax: (208) 745-0212

Illinois	Chicago	Dermatologist	Garden, Jerome M. MD 150 East Huron Street Suite 910 Chicago, IL 60611 Phone: (312) 280-0890 Fax: (312) 208-9615
Illinois	Chicago	Dermatologist	Jacob, Carolyn MD Chicago Cosmetic Surgery and Dermatology 20 W. Kinze Street Suite 1130 Chicago, IL (312) 245-9965 www.chicagodermatology.com
Illinois	Chicago	Dermatologist	Taub, Amy MD 275 Parkway Drive Lincolnshire, IL 60069 Phone: (847) 459-6400 www.advdermatology.com
Illinois	Chicago	Dermatologist	Murad, Alam MD Northwestern University Dermatology 675 N. St. Clair 19-150 Chicago, IL 60611 Phone: (312) 695-6647 Fax: (312) 695-0529 m-alam@northwestern.edu
Iowa	Iowa City	Dermatologist	Arpey, Christopher J. MD Department of Dermatology University of Iowa Hospitals 200 Hawkins Drive Iowa City, IA 52242 Phone: (319) 356-2856
Louisiana	Kenner	Dermatologist	Farber, George A. MD Gulf South Medical and Surgical Institute, Incorporated 3705 Florida Avenue Kenner, LA 70065 Phone: (504) 471-3100

Maryland	Hunt Valley	Dermatologist	Weiss, Robert A. MD
			54 Scott Adam Road
			Suite 302
			Hunt Valley, MD 21030
			Phone: 410-666-3960
			Fax: 410-666-0203
			rweiss@mdlsv.com
Massachusetts	Boston	Dermatologist	Anderson, R. Rox MD
			Massachusetts General Hospital
			Department of Dermatology
			Wellman Laboratories
			55 Fruit Street
			Boston, MA 02114
			Phone: (617) 726- 6168
			Fax: (617) 726- 6121
			bdammin@partners.org
Massachusetts	Boston	Dermatologist	Manstein, Dieter MD
			Wellman Center for Photomedicine
			50 Blossom Street, BXH 630
			Boston, MA 02114
			Phone: (617) 726-4893
			Fax: (617) 724-2075
			dmanstein@partners.org
Massachusetts	Boston/ Chestnut Hill	Dermatologist	Arndt, Kenneth MD.
			Dover, Jeffrey S. MD FRCPC
			Kaminer, Michael S. MD
			Rohrer, Thomas E. MD
			Skin Care Physicians of Chestnut Hill
			1244 Boylston Street (Route 9)
			Chestnut Hill, MA
			Phone: (617) 731-1600
			Fax: (617) 731-1601
			www.skincarephysicians.net
			jdover@skincarephysicians.net
			mkaminer@skincarephysicians.net
			trohrer@skincarephysicians.net

Michigan	Ann Arbor	Dermatologist	Orringer, Jeffrey MD University of Michigan 1500 E. Medical Center Drive Ann Arbor, MI 48109 Phone: (734) 923-3377 Fax: (734) 936-6395 jorringe@umich.edu
Michigan	Ypsilanti	Dermatologist	Boyd, Charles MD Gillard, Montgomery MD The Boyd Gillard Institute of Aesthetic & Dermatologic Surgery 4990 W. Clark Road Building A, Suite 200 Ypsilanti, MI 48197 Phone: (734) 572-7500 Fax: (734) 572-7777 www.ihacares.com
Minnesota	Minneapolis	Dermatologist	Zelickson, Brian D. MD 1002 Medical Arts Building 825 Nicollet Mall Minneapolis, MN 55405 Phone: (612) 338-0711 Fax: (612)332-3663 Zelic002@earthlink.net
Missouri	Saint Louis	Dermatologist	Hruza, George MD Laser and Dermatologic Surgery Center 14377 Woodlake Drive Suite 111 Chesterfield, MO 63017 Phone: (314) 878-3839 Fax: (314)878-6575 ghruza@aol.com www.lasersurgeryusa.com
Missouri	Saint Louis	Dermatologist	Glaser, Dee Anna MD Saint Louis University Department of Dermatology 2325 Dougherty Ferry Road Suite 102 Saint Louis, MO 63122 Phone: (314) 977-9666 http://dermatology.slu.edu/

Nebraska	Omaha	Dermatologist	Schlessinger, Joel MD
			Skin Specialists PC
			2802 Oak View Mall Drive
			Omaha, NE 68144
			Phone: (402) 334-SKIN (7546)
			Toll-free: (800) 757-7546
			Fax: 402.334.8627
			www.lovelyskin.com
Nevada	Las Vegas	Dermatologist	Safko, Martin MD
			311 N. Buffalo
			Suite A
			Las Vegas, NV 89128
			Phone: (702) 731-0933
			www.southwestdermatology.com
Nevada	Las Vegas	Dermatologist	Michaels, Jason MD
			Aspire Cosmetic MedCenter
			9097 W. Post Rd, Suite 110
			Las Vegas, NV 89148
			Phone: (702) 588-7447
			www.aspiremedcenter.com
New York	New York	Dermatologist	Brandt, Fred MD
			317 E. Thirty-fourth Street
			6th Floor
			New York, NY 10016
			Phone (212) 889-7096
			Fax (212) 686-0097
			www.drbrandtskincare.com
New York	New York	Dermatologist	Geronemus, Roy G. MD
			Laser and Skin Surgery Center of NY
			317 East Thirty-fourth Street
			Suite 11 North
			New York, NY 10016
			Phone: (212) 686-7306
			Fax: (212) 686-7305
			mail@laserskinsurgery.com
New York	New York	Dermatologist	Polis, Laurie J. MD
			62 Crosby Street
			New York, NY 10012-4410
			Phone: (212) 431-1600
			Fax: (212) 431-7521
			drpolis@sohoderm.com

New York	New York	Dermatologist	Grossman, Melanie C. MD 161 Madison Avenue, 4 NW New York, NY 10016 Phone: (212) 725-8600 Fax: (212) 725-8620 mgrossmanmd@earthlink.net
New York	New York	Dermatologist	Katz, Bruce MD Juva Skin and Laser Center 60 East Fifty-sixth Street New York, NY 10002 Phone: (212) 688-5882 Fax: (212) 421-9502 brukatz@juvaskin.com
New York	New York	Dermatologist	Kauvar, Arielle N.B. MD New York Laser and Skin Center 1044 Fifth Avenue New York, NY 10028 Phone: (212) 249-9440 Fax: (212) 249-9441 drkauvar@hotmail.com
New York	New York	Dermatologist	Wexler, Patricia MD. Wexler Dermatology, P.C. 145 East Thirty-second Street New York, NY 10016 Phone: (212) 684-2626 Fax: (212) 684-6906 www.patriciawexlermd.com
New York	New York	Dermatologist	Cook-Bolden, Fran MD 20 East Sixty-sixth Street Suite 1A New York, NY 10021 Phone: (212) 249-8377 Fax: (212) 249-8372 www.cookboldenskinandlaser.com
New York	White Plains	Dermatologist	Narins, Rhoda MD Dermatology Surgery and Laser Center 222 Westchester Ave. White Plains, NY 10604 (212) 288-9910

North Carolina	Chapel Hill	Dermatologist	Cox, Sue Ellen MD Aesthetic Solutions 5821 Farrington Road Suite 101 Chapel Hill, NC 27517 Phone: (919) 403-6200 www.aesthetic-solutions.com
North Carolina	High Point	Dermatologist	Draelos, Zoe MD 2444 North Main Street High Point, NC 27262 Phone: (336) 841-2040
Oklahoma	Edmond	Dermatologist	John, Michael MD Edmond Dermatology Center 620 West Fifteenth Street Edmond, OK 73013 Phone: (405) 359-0551 Contact: Reba (wife)
Oklahoma	Tulsa	Dermatologist	Alexander, Jeff MD. 6565 South Yale Avenue Suite 110 Tulsa, OK 74136 Phone: (918) 494-8304 Contact: Judy (wife) www.skincareinstitute.net
Oregon	Portland	Dermatologist	Klein, Marla MD Klein Dermatology & Associates 9495 Southwest Locust Street Suite A Portland, OR 97223 (503) 445-2200 http://kleindermatology.com
Pennsylvania	Bryn Mawr	Dermatologist	Bernstein, Eric F. MD Main Line Center for Laser Surgery 931 Haverford Road Bryn Mawr, PA 19010 Phone: (610) 581-7400 Fax: (610) 581-0568 dermguy@hotmail.com

Pennsylvania	Philadelphia	Dermatologist	Greenbaum, Steven MD Skin and Laser Surgery Center 1528 Walnut Street Suite 1101 Philadelphia, PA 19102 Phone: (213) 735-4994
Tennessee	Nashville	Dermatologist	Biesman, Brian J. MD 345 Twenty-third Avenue North Suite 416 Nashville, TN 37203 Phone: (615) 329-1110 Fax: (615) 320-0192 bbies@mindspring.com
Tennessee	Nashville	Dermatologist	Gold, Michael H. MD Gold Skin Care Center 2000 Richard Jones Road Nashville, TN 37215-2885 Phone: (615) 383-2400 Fax: (615) 385-0387 www.goldskincare.com
Texas	Houston	Dermatologist	Bruce, Suzanne MD 1900 St. James Place Suite 650 Houston, TX 77056 Phone: (713) 850-0240 www.sba-skincare.com
Vermont	Burlington	Dermatologist	Goldman, Glenn MD Fletcher Allen Health Care Dermatology Division 1 South Prospect Street Burlington, VT 05401-3498 Phone: (802) 847-0761 www.fahc.org
Washington	Kirkland	Dermatologist	Cooperrider, Peter MD Evergreen Professional Plaza 12911 120th Avenue NE Suite G-100 Kirkland, WA 98034 Phone: (425) 899-4144 Fax: (425) 899-4148 www.kirklandlaser.com

Washington	Kirkland	Dermatologist	Voss, Julie E. MD 3100 Carillon Point Kirkland, WA 98033 Phone: (425) 576-1700 10330 Meridian Avenue N Suite 240 Seattle, WA 98134 Phone: (206) 525-2525 www.nwface.com
Washington	Bellevue		Bauman, Carla MD Bellevue Dermatology Clinic 1260 116th Avenue NE Bellevue, WA Phone: (425) 455-3376
Washington	Seattle	Dermatologist	Irwin, Brandith MD 1101 Madison Street, Suite 1490 Seattle, WA 98104–3598 Phone: (206) 215-6600 Fax: (206) 215-6650 frontdesk@madisonkin.com
Washington	Spokane	Dermatologist	Werschler, Philip W. MD 104 West Fifth Avenue Suite 330 Spokane, WA 99204 Phone: (509) 624-1184 Fax: (509) 921-7144 www.spokanederm.com

INTERNATIONAL

Canada	Montreal	Dermatologist	Barolet, Daniel MD McGill University 3333 Graham Boulevard Suite 206 Montreal, H3R 3L5 Canada Phone: (514) 343-4444 Fax: (514) 344-8258 dbarolet@opusmed.com

Canada	Ontario	Dermatologist	Smith, Kevin C. MD FRCPC Niagra Falls Dermatology & Skin Care Center 6453 Morrison Street Suite 201 Niagra Falls, ON L2E 7H1 Canada ksmithderm@gmail.com
Canada	Vancouver	Dermatologist	Carruthers, Alastair MD Carruthers Dermatology Center Inc. 943 West Broadway, Suite 820 Vancouver, BC V5Z 4E1 Canada Phone: (604) 714-0222 Fax: (604) 714-0223 alastair@carruthers.net
China`	Hong Kong	Dermatologist	Chan, Henry H.L. MD Thirteenth Floor, Club Lusitano 16 Ice House Street Central Hong Kong, China Phone: +852-210-99999 Fax: +852-210-99993 Corrinne@hhlchan.com
England	London	Dermatologist	Lowe, Nicholas, MD The Cranley Clinic 3 Harcourt House, 19A Cavendish Square London W1G 0PN Phone: 020-7499-3223 Fax: 020-7499-1101 cranleyuk@aol.com
Germany	Regensburg	Dermatologist	Szeimes, Rolf-Markus, MD PhD Regensburg University Hospital Franz-Josef-Strauss-Allee 11 Regensburg, Germany D-93053 Phone: +49-941-944-9614 Fax: +49-941-944-9628 Rolf-markus.szeimes@ klinik.uni-regensburg.de

| Switzerland | Geneva | Dermatologist | Adatto, Maurice A. MD
SKINPULSE Dermatology Center
5 Rd. Pt Plainpalais
Geneva, CH-1205
Phone: +41-22-329-7000
Fax: +41-22-320-8088
madatto@skinpulse.ch |

REFERENCES

CHAPTER 1

Baumann, L. *The Skin-Type Solution.* New York: Bantam Dell, 2006.

Begoun, P. *Don't Go to the Cosmetics Counter Without Me.* Seattle: Beginning Press, 2003.

Bissett, D. L., J. E. Oblong, et al. "Niacinamide: A B Vitamin that Improves Aging Facial Skin Appearance." *Dermatol Surg* 31:7 (2005): 860–5.

Brown, Bobbi. *Bobbi Brown Beauty: The Ultimate Beauty Resource.* Scarborough, ON: Harper Collins, 1998.

Kameyama, K., C. Sakai, et al. "Inhibitory Effect of Magnesium L-Ascorbyl–2-Phosphate (VC-PMG) on Melanogenesis In Vitro and In Vivo." *J Am Acad Dermatol* 34 (1996): 29–33.

Chiu, A. E., J. L. Chan, et al. "Double Blinded, Placebo Controlled Trial of Green Tea Extracts in the Clinical and Histologic Appearance of Photoaging Skin." *Dermatol Surg* 31:7 (2005): 855–860.

Consumer Reports, January 2007.

Dahiya, A., J. Romano. "Cosmeceuticals: A Review of Their Use for Aging and Photoaged Skin." *Cosm Derm* 19 (2006): 479–484.

Darr, D., S. Combs, S. Pinnell, et al. "Topical Vitamin C Protects Porcine Skin From Ultraviolet Radiation-Induced Damage." *Brit J Derm* 127 (1992): 247–53.

Darr, D., S. Dunston, H. Faust, et al. "Effectiveness of Antioxidants (Vitamin C and E) With and Without Sunscreens as Topical Photoprotectants." *Acta Derm Venereol* 76 (1996): 264–8.

Darvin, M., L. Zastrow, W. Sterry, et al. "Effect of Supplemented and Topically Applied Antioxidant Substances on Human Tissue." *Skin Pharmacol Physiol* 19(5) (2006): 238–47.

Fitzpatrick, R. E. "Endogenous Growth Factors as Cosmeceuticals." *Dermatol Surg* 31 (2005): 827–31.

Griffiths, C. M., A. N. Russman, et al. "Restoration of Collagen Formation in Photodamaged Human Skin by Tretinoin." *New Engl J Med* 329 (1993): 530–5.

Keri, J., and L. Baumann. "The Science Behind Vitamin C." *Skin & Aging* (1999): 79–80.

Lupo, M. P. "Cosmeceutical Peptides." *Dermatol Surg* 31:7 (2005): 832–6.

Podda, M., and M. Grundmann-Kollmann. "Low Molecular Weight Antioxidants and Their Role in Skin Aging." *Clin Exp Dermatol* October 26 (7) (2001): 578–82.

Kligman, A. M., G. L. Grove, et al. "Topical Tretinoin for Photoaged Skin." *J Am Acad Dermatol* 615 (1986): 836–9.

Schwartz, J. R., Z. D. Draelos, et al. "Zinc and Skin Health: Overview of Physiology and Pharmacology." *Dermatol Surg* 31:7 (2005): 837–47.

Thiele, J. J., S. N. Hsieh, et al. "Vitamin E: Critical Review of Its Current Use in Cosmetic and Clinical Dermatology." *Dermatol Surg* 31:7 (2005): 805–13.

Thornfeldt, C. "Cosmeceuticals Containing Herbs: Fact, Fiction and Future." *Dermatol Surg* 31:7 (2005): 873–80.

CHAPTER 3

Born, T. "Hyaluronic Acid." *Clin Plas Surg* 33 (2006): 525–538.

Carruthers, J. A., and J. D. Carruthers. "Botulinum Toxin Type-A Treatment of Multiple Upper Facial Sites: Patient-Reported Outcomes." *Dermatol Surg* 33 (2007): S10–S17.

Carruthers, J. A., and J. D. Carruthers. "Treatment of Glabellar Frown Lines with C. Botulinum-A Exotoxin." *J Dermatol Surg Oncol* 18 (1992):17–21.

Carruthers, J. A., and J. D. Carruthers. "Eyebrow Height After Botulinum-A to the Glabella." *Dermatol Surg* 33 (2007): S26–S31.

Carruthers, J. D., N. J. Lowe, M. A. Menter, et al. "Double-Blind, Placebo—Controlled Study of the Safety and Efficacy of Botulinum Toxin Type-A for Patients with Glabellar Lines." *Plast Reconstr Surg* 112 (2003):1089–98.

Sadick, N., and L. Sorhaindo. "The Cosmetic Use of Botulinum Type-B." *INT Ophthalmol Clin* 45 (2005):153–61.

CHAPTER 4

Biesman, B. S., S. S. Baker, J. Carruthers, et al. "Monopolar Radiofrequency Treatment of Human Eyelids: A Prospective, Multicenter, Efficacy Trial." *Lasers Surg Med* 38 (2006): 890–8.

Kane, M. "Classification of Crow's Feet Patterns Among Caucasian Women: The Key to Individualizing Treatment." *Plast Reconst Surg* 112 (2003): 33S–39S.

Kane, M. A. "Treatment of Tear-Trough Deformity and Lower-Lid Bowing with Injectable Hyaluronic Acid." *Aesth Plast Surg* 29 (2005): 363–7.

Carruthers, J. A., and J. D. Carruthers. "Botulinum Toxin Type-A Treatment of Multiple Upper Facial Sites: Patient-Reported Outcomes." *Dermatol Surg* 33 (2007): S10–S17.

Carruthers, J., S. Faggien, S. L. Matarasso, and Botox Consensus Group. "Consensus Recommendations on the Use of Botulinum Toxin Type A in Facial Aesthetics." *Plast Reconstr Surg* 114 (suppl.) (2004): 1S–22S.

Elder, J. A. "Ocular Effects of Radiofrequency Energy." *Bioelectromagnetics Supplement* 6 (2003): S148–S161.

Garcia, A., Fulton, J. E. Jr. "Cosmetic Denervation of the Muscles of Facial Expression with Botulinum Toxin: A Dose Response Study." *Dermatol Surg* 22 (1996): 39–43.

Goldberg, D. J., and J. A. Samady. "Intense Pulsed Light and Nd: YAG Laser Non-ablative Treatment of Facial Rhytides." *Lasers Surg Med* 28 (2001): 141–4.

Lupton, J. R., C. M. Williams, and T. S. Alster. "Non-Ablative Laser Skin Resurfacing Using a 1,540-nm Erbium Glass Laser: A Clinical and Histologic Analysis." *Dermatol Surg* 28 (2002): 833–5.

Tanzi, E. L., C. M. Williams, and T. S. Alster. "Treatment of Facial Rhytides with a Non-Ablative 1,450-nm Diode Laser: A Controlled Clinical and Histologic Study." *Dermatol Surg* 29 (2003): 124–8.

CHAPTER 5

Avram, D. K., and M. P. Goldman. "The Safety and Effectiveness of Single Pass Erbium:YAG Laser in the Treatment of Mild to Moderate Photodamage." *Dermatol Surg* 30 (2004): 1073–6.

Fisher, G. H., and R. G. Geronemus. "Short-Term Side Effects of Fractional Photothermolysis." *Dermatol Surg* 31 (2005): 1245–9.

Fisher, G., L. Jacobson, L. Bernstein, et al. "Non-Ablative Radiofrequency Treatment of Facial Laxity." *Dermatol Surg* 31 (2005): 1237–41.

Fitzpatrick, R. E., M. P. Goldman, et al. "Pulsed Carbon Dioxide Laser Resurfacing of Photo Aged Skin." *Arch Dermatol* 132 (1996): 395–402.

Fitzpatrick, R., R. Geronemus, D. Goldberg, et al. "Multicenter Study of Noninvasive Radiofrequency for Periorbital Tissue Tightening." *Lasers Surg Med* 33 (2003): 232–42.

Fritz, M., J. T. Counters, and B. D. Zelickson. "Radiofrequency Treatment for Middle and Lower Face Laxity." *Arch Facial Plast Surg* 6 (2004): 370–3.

Geronemus, R. G. "Fractional Photothermolysis: Current and Future Applications." *Lasers Surg Med* 38 (2006): 169–76.

Goldberg, D. J., and J. A. Samady. "Intense Pulsed Light and Nd: YAG Laser Non-ablative Treatment of Facial Rhytides." *Lasers Surg Med* 28 (2001): 141–4.

Iyer, S., R. E. Fitzpatrick, et al. "Using a Radiofrequency Energy Device to Treat the Lower Face: A Treatment Paradigm for a Nonsurgical Facelift." *Cosmet Dermatol* 16 (2003): 37–40.

Levy, J. L., M. Trelles, et al. "Treatment of Wrinkles with the Non-Ablative 1,320-nm Nd: YAG Laser." *Ann Plast Surg* 47 (2001): 482–8.

Lupton, J. R., C. M. Williams, and T. S. Alster. "Non-Ablative Laser Skin Resurfacing Using a 1,540-nm Erbium Glass Laser: A Clinical and Histologic Analysis." *Dermatol Surg* 28 (2002): 833–5.

Manstein, D., G. S. Herron, R. K. Sink, et al. "Fractional Photothermolysis: A New Concept for Cutaneous Remodeling Using Microscopic Patterns of Thermal Injury." *Laser Surg Med* 34 (2004): 426–38.

Narins, D. J., and R. S. Narins. "Nonsurgical Radiofrequency Facelift." *J Drugs Dermatol* 2 (2003): 495–500.

Tanzi, E. L., C. M. Williams, T. S. Alster. "Treatment of Facial Rhytides with a Non-Ablative 1,450-nm Diode Laser: A Controlled Clinical and Histologic Study." *Dermatol Surg* 29 (2003): 124–8.

Valantin, M., C. Aubron-Olivier, et al. "Poly-Lactic Acid Implants to Correct Facial Lipoatrophy in HIV-Infected Patients: Results of an Open Label Study VEGA." *AIDS* 17 (2003): 2471–7.

Vleggar, D. "Facial Volumetric Correction with Injectable Poly-L-Lactic-Acid." *Dermatol Surg* 31 (2005): 1511–8

Vleggar, D., and U. Bauer. "Facial Enhancement and the European Experience with Sculptra (Poly-L-Lactic-Acid)." *J Drugs Dermatol* 3 (2004): 542–7.

Wanner, M., E. Tanzi, and T. Alster. "Fractional Photothermolysis Treatment of Facial and Nonfacial Cutaneous Photo Damage With a 1,550-nm Erbium-Doped Fiber Laser." *Dermatol Surg* 33 (2007): 23–8.

Woerle, B., C. W. Hanke, et al. "Poly-L-Lactic Acid: A Temporary Filler for Soft Tissue Augmentation." *J Drugs Dermatol* 3 (2004): 385–9.

CHAPTER 6

Engelman, D. E., B. Bloom, and D. J. Goldberg. "Dermal Fillers: Complications and Informed Consent." *J Cosmet Laser Ther* 7 (2005):29–32.

Dover, J. S., and B. Zelickson. "Results of a 5,700 Patient Monopolar Radiofrequency Facial Skin Tightening Treatments: Assessment of a Low-Energy Multiple-Pass Technique Leading to a Clinical End Point Algorithm." *Dermatol Surg* 33 (2007): 900–7.

Friedman, P. M., E. A. Mafong, A.N. Kauvar, et al. "Safety Data of Injectable Non-animal Stabilized Hyaluronic Acid Gel for Soft Tissue Augmentation." *Dermatol Surg* 28 (2002): 491–4.

Goldman, M. P., T. S. Alster, and R. Weiss. "A Randomized Trial to Determine the Influence of Laser Therapy, Monopolar Radiofrequency Treatment and Intense Pulsed Light Therapy Administered Immediately After Hyaluronic Acid Gel Implantation." *Dermatol Surg* 33 (2007): 535–42.

Sadick, N. S. "Soft Tissue Augmentation: Selection, Mode of Operation, and Proper Use of Injectable Agents." *Cosmet Dermatol* 20 (suppl. 2) (2007): 8–13.

Sklar, J., and S. M. White. "Radiance FN: A New Soft Tissue Filler." *Dermatol Surg* 30 (2004): 764–8.

CHAPTER 7

Dover, J. S., and B. Zelickson. "Results of a 5,700 Patient Monopolar Radiofrequency Facial Skin Tightening Treatments: Assessment of a Low-Energy Multiple-Pass Technique Leading to a Clinical End Point Algorithm." *Dermatol Surg* 33 (2007):900–7.

Fisher, G., L. Jacobson, L. Bernstein, et al. "Nonablative Radiofrequency Treatment of Facial Laxity." *Dermatol Surg* 31 (2005): 1237–41.

Fitzpatrick, R., R. Geronemus, D. Goldberg, et al. "Multicenter Study of Noninvasive Radiofrequency for Periorbital Tissue Tightening." *Lasers Surg Med* 33 (2003): 232–42.

Fritz, M., J. T. Counters, and B. D. Zelitkson. "Radiofrequency Treatment for Middle and Lower Face Laxity." *Arch Facial Plast Surg* 6 (2004): 370–3.

Iyer, S., R. E. Fitzpatrick, et al. "Using a Radiofrequency Energy Device to Treat the Lower Face: A Treatment Paradigm for a Nonsurgical Facelift." *Cosmet Dermatol* 16 (2003): 37–40.

Levy, J. L., M. Trelles, et al. "Treatment of Wrinkles with the Nonablative 1,320-nm Nd: YAG Laser." *Ann Plast Surg* 47 (2001): 482–8.

Narins, D. J., and R. S. Narins. "Nonsurgical Radiofrequency Facelift." *J Drug Dermatol* 2 (2003): 495–500.

Sadick, N. S. "Soft Tissue Augmentation: Selection, Mode of Operation, and Proper Use of Injectable Agents." *Cosmet Dermatol* 20 (suppl. 2) (2007): 8–13.

Tanzi, E. L., C. M. Williams, T. S. Alster. "Treatment of Facial Rhytides with a Non-Ablative 1,450-nm Diode Laser: A Controlled Clinical and Histologic Study." *Dermatol Surg* 29 (2003): 124–8.

Valantin, M., C. Aubron-Olivier, et al. "Poly-Lactic Acid Implants to Correct Facial Lipoatrophy in HIV-Infected Patients: Results of an Open Label Study VEGA." *AIDS* 17:17 (2003): 2471–7.

Vleggar, D. "Facial Volumetric Correction with Injectable Poly-L-Lactic-Acid." *Dermatol Surg* 31 (2005): 1511–8.

Vleggar, D., and U. Bauer. "Facial Enhancement and the European Experience with Sculptra (Poly-L-Lactic-Acid)." *J Drugs Dermatol* 3 (2004): 542–7.

Woerle, B., C. W. Hanke, et al. "Poly-L-Lactic Acid: A Temporary Filler for Soft Tissue Augmentation." *J Drugs Dermatol* 3 (2004): 385–9.

CHAPTER 8

Alster, T. S., and E. Tanzi. "Improvement of Neck and Cheek Laxity with a Nonablative Radiofrequency Device: A Lifting Experience." *Dermatol Surg* 30 (2004): 503–7.

Bitter, P. H. "Noninvasive Rejuvenation of Photodamaged Skin Using Serial, Full-Face Intense Pulsed Light Treatments." *Dermatol Surg* 26 (2000): 835–43.

Kane, M. A. "Nonsurgical Treatment of Platysmal Bands with Injection of Botulinum Toxin A." *Plast Reconstr Surg* 103 (1999): 656–63.

Fisher, G. H., R. G. Geronemus. "Short-Term Side Effects of Fractional Photothermolysis." *Dermatol Surg* 31 (2005): 1245–9.

Gold, M. H. "Intense Pulsed Light Therapy for Photorejuvenation Enhanced with 20% Aminolevulinic Acid Photodynamic Therapy." *J Lasers Med Surg* 15 (suppl.) (2003): 47.

Goldberg, D. "New Collagen Formation After Dermal Remodeling with an Intense Pulsed Light Source." *J Cutan Laser Ther* 2 (2000): 59–61.

Goldberg, D. J., and K. B. Cutler. "Nonablative Treatment of Rhytides with Intense Pulsed Light." *Lasers Surg Med* 26 (2000): 196–200.

Kawada, A., and H. Shiraishi, et al. "Clinical Improvement of Solar Lentigines and Ephelides with an Intense Pulsed Light Source." *Dermatol Surg* 28 (2002): 504–8.

Manstein, D., G. S. Herron, R. K. Sink, et al. "Fractional Photothermolysis: A New Concept for Cutaneous Remodeling Using Microscopic Patterns of Thermal Injury." *Laser Surg Med* 34 (2004): 426–38.

Narurkar, V. "To Ablate, Non-Ablate or Fractionate: Realities Versus Hype in Deviced-Based Aesthetic Medicine." *Cosm Derm* 19 (2006): 349–53.

Ortonne, J. P., A. Pandya, et al. "Treatment of Solar Lentigines." *J Am Acad Dermatol* 54 (2006): S262–S271.

Touma, D., M. Yaar, et al. "A Trial of Short Incubation, Broad-Area Photodynamic Therapy for Facial Actinic Keratoses and Diffuse Photodamage." *Arch Dermatol* 140 (2004): 33–40.

Wanner, M., E. Tanzi, and T. Alster. "Fractional Photothermolysis Treatment of Facial and Nonfacial Cutaneous Photo Damage with a 1,550-nm Erbium-Doped Fiber Laser." *Dermatol Surg* 33 (2007): 23–8.

Weiss, R. A., M. P. Goldman, et al. "Treatment of Poikiloderma of Civatte with an Intense Pulsed Light Source." *Dermatol Surg* 26 (2000): 823–8.

Zelickson, B., D. KiStreet "Effect of Pulsed Dye Laser and Intense Pulsed Light Source on the Dermal Extracellular Matrix Remodeling." *Laser Surg Med Suppl* 12 (2000): 17.

Chapter 9

Alam, M., J. S. Dover, and K. A. Arndt. "Treatment of Facial Telangiectasias with Variable-Pulse High-Fluence Pulsed-Dye Laser: Comparison of Efficacy with Fluences Immediately Above and Below the Purpura Threshold." *Dermatol Surg* 29 (2003): 681–5.

Bitter, P. H. "Noninvasive Rejuvenation of Photodamaged Skin Using Serial, Full-Face Intense Pulsed Light Treatments." *Dermatol Surg* 26 (2000): 835–43.

Coleman, W. P., and H. J. Brodie. "Advances in Chemical Peeling." *Dermatol Clin* 15 (1997): 19–26.

Conde, J. F., S. R. Feldman, et al. "Managing Rosacea: A Review of Use of Metronidazol Alone and in Combination with Oral Antibiotics." *J Drug Dermatol* 6 (2007): 495–98.

Dahl, M. V., H. I. Katz, G. G. Krueger, et al. "Topical Metronidazol Maintains Remissions of Rosacea." *Arch Dermatol* 134 (1998): 679–83.

Goldberg, D. "New Collagen Formation After Dermal Remodeling with an Intense Pulsed Light Source." *J Cutan Laser Ther* 2 (2000): 59–61.

Keeling, J., L. Cardona, et al. "Combining Topical Therapy with Procedures to Treat Hyper-pigmentation Disorders." *Cosm Derm* 20 (2007): 223–7.

Kawada, A., and H. Shiraishi, et al. "Clinical Improvement of Solar Lentigines and Ephelides with an Intense Pulsed Light Source." *Dermatol Surg* 28 (2002): 504–8.

Ortonne, J. P., A. Pandya, et al. "Treatment of Solar Lentigines." *J Am Acad Dermatol* 54 (2006): S262–S271.

Nally, J., and D. S. Berson. "Topical Therapies for Rosacea." *J Drug Dermatol* 5 (2006): 23–6.

Pathak, M. A., T. B. Fitzpatrick, et al. "Usefulness of Retinoic Acid in the Treatment of Melasma." *J Am Acad Dermatol* 15 (1986): 894–9.

Rokhsar, C. K., Y. Tse, R. E. Fitzpatrick. "The Treatment of Melasma with Fractional Photothermolysis: A Pilot Study." *Dermatol Surg* 31 (2005): 1645–50.

Sharquie, K. E., M. M. Al-Tikreety, et al. "Lactic Acid Chemical Peels as a New Therapeutic Modality in Melasma in Comparison to Jessner's Solution Chemical Peels." *Dermatol Surg* 32 (2006): 1429–36.

Tannous, Z. S., and S. Astner. "Utilizing Fractional Resurfacing in the Treatment of Therapy-Resistant Melasma." *J Cosmet Laser Ther* 7 (2005): 39–43.

Weiss, R. A., M. P. Goldman, et al. "Treatment of Poikiloderma of Civatte with an Intense Pulsed Light Source." *Dermatol Surg* 26 (2000): 823–8.

West, T. B., and T. S. Alster. "Comparison of the Long-Pulse Dye (590–595 nm) and KTP (532-nm) Lasers in the Treatment of Facial and Leg Telangiectasias." *Dermatol Surg* 24 (1998): 221–6.

Zelickson, B., D. Kist. "Effect of Pulsed Dye Laser and Intense Pulsed Light Source on the Dermal Extracellular Matrix Remodeling." *Laser Surg Med Suppl* 12 (2000): 17.

CHAPTER 13

Giampapa, Vincent. *The Basic Principles and Practice of Anti-aging Medicine & Age Management for the Aesthetic Surgeon and Physician.* Vincent Giampapa, 2003.

Pratt, Steven. *SuperFoods Rx: 14 Foods That Will Change Your Life.* New York: HarperCollins, 2005.

Roisen, M. F., and M. C. Oz. *You: The Owner's Manual An Insider's Guide to the Body that Will Make You Healthier and Younger.* New York: HarperCollins, 2005.

Stahl, W., U. Heinrich, et al. "Lycopine Rich Products and Dietary Photoprotection." *Photochem Photobiol Sci* 5 (2006): 238–42.

Stahl, W., and H. Sies. "Bioactivity and Protective Effects of Natural Carotenoids." *Biochim Biophys Acta* May 30 1740 (2) (2005): 101–7.

Thirunavukkarasu, V., et al. "Fructose Diet-Induced Skin Collagen Abnormalities Are Prevented by Lipoic Acid." *Exp Diabesity Res* 5 (4) (2004): 237–44.

CHAPTER 14

Miquel, J, A. Ramirez-Bosca, et al. "Menopause: A Review on the Role of Oxygen Stress and Favorable Effects of Dietary Antioxidants." *Arch Gerontol Geriatr* May 42 (3) (2006): 289–306.

Raine-Fenning N. J., M. P. Brincat. "Skin Aging and Menopause: Implications for Treatment." *Am J Clin Dermatol* 4(6) (2003): 371–8.

Sator P. G., J. B. Schmidt, et al. "The Influence of Hormone Replacement Therapy on Skin Aging: A Pilot Study." *Maturitas* 39 (1) (July 25, 2001):43–55.

Shah M. G., H. I. Maibach. "Estrogen and Skin. An Overview." *Am J Clin Dermatol* 2(3) (2001):143–50.

CHAPTER 16

American Society for Dermatologic Surgery. *Guidelines for Ethical Patient Safety Practices.* 2007.

CHAPTER 17

Amin, S. P., D. J. Goldberg, et al. "Mesotherapy for Facial Skin Rejuvenation: A Clinical, Histologic, and Electron Microscopic Evaluation." *Dermatol Surg* 32 (2006): 1467–72.

Fisher, G. H., R. G. Geronemus. "Short-Term Side Effects of Fractional Photothermolysis." *Dermatol Surg* 31 (2005): 1245–9.

Geronemus, R. G. "Fractional Photothermolysis: Current and Future Applications." *Lasers Surg Med* 38 (2006): 169–76.

Gold, M. H. "Intense Pulsed Light Therapy for Photorejuvenation Enhanced with 20% Aminolevulinic Acid Photodynamic Therapy." *J Lasers Med Surg* 15 (suppl.) (2003): 47.

Laubach, H., R. Anderson, D. Manstein, et al. "Skin Responses to Fractional Photothermolysis." *Laser Surg Med* 38 (2006): 142–9.

Mack, J. "Nanotechnology: What's In It for Biotech?" *Biotechnology Healthcare* December (2005): 29–36.

Manstein, D., G. S. Herron, R. K. Sink, et al. "Fractional Photothermolysis: A New Concept for Cutaneous Remodeling Using Microscopic Patterns of Thermal Injury." *Laser Surg Med* 34 (2004): 426–38.

Rotunda, A. M., and M. S. Kolodney. "Mesotherapy and Phosphatidylcholine Injections: Historical Clarification and Review." *Dermatol Surg* 32 (2006): 465–80.

Ruiz-Rodriquez, R., et al. "Photodynamic Photorejuvenation." *Dermatol Surg* 28 (2002): 742–4.

Touma, D., M. Yaar, et al. "A Trial of Short Incubation, Broad-Area Photodynamic Therapy for Facial Actinic Keratoses and Diffuse Photodamage." *Arch Dermatol* 140 (2004): 33–40.

Wanner, M., E. Tanzi, and T. Alster. "Fractional Photothermolysis Treatment of Facial and Nonfacial Cutaneous Photo Damage With a 1,550-nm Erbium-Doped Fiber Laser." *Dermatol Surg* 33 (2007): 23–8.

INDEX